Conquer Your Pain in 9 Steps

Library and Archives Canada Cataloguing in Publication

Staveley, Carole, 1965-, author
    Conquer your pain in 9 steps : building the mindset and team you need to suffer less and achieve more / Carole Staveley.

Includes bibliographical references.
Issued in print and electronic formats.
ISBN 978-1-77141-114-1 (pbk.).--ISBN 978-1-77141-115-8 (html)

    1. Chronic pain--Popular works. 2. Chronic pain--Psychological aspects--Popular works. 3. Chronic pain--Prevention--Popular works. 4. Self-care, Health--Popular works. I. Title.

RB127.S73 2015   616'.0472   C2015-901222-8
                                                 C2015-901223-6

Conquer Your Pain in 9 Steps

Building the Mindset and Team You Need to Suffer Less and Achieve More

Carole Staveley

Book Cover Design: Trista Baldwin
Editor: Nina Shoroplova
Assistant Editor: Susan Kehoe
Production Editor: Jennifer Kaleta
Typeset: Greg Salisbury
Portrait Photographer: TNy Photography

DISCLAIMER: The information provided in this book is designed to be an educational aid only. It is not intended in any way to replace other professional healthcare or mental health advice, nor is it intended to be used for medical diagnosis or treatment. If you suspect that you have a medical condition, always consult your healthcare provider. Readers of this publication agree that neither Carole Staveley nor her publisher will be held responsible or liable for damages that may be alleged or resulting, directly or indirectly, from their use of this publication. All external links are provided as a resource only and are not guaranteed to remain active for any length of time. Neither the publisher nor the author can be held accountable for the information provided by, or actions resulting from accessing these resources.

Special Note: The term IRONMAN® is a registered trademark of World Triathlon Corporation. When used in this book, it refers specifically to full distance triathlon races sanctioned by World Triathlon Corporation. A full distance triathlon is an event involving a 3.8 km (2.4 miles) swim, 180 km (112 miles) of cycling, and a 42.2 km (26.2 miles) run, in that order. The author is not affiliated with nor does she represent World Triathlon Corporation.

For my husband, Rod—My unconditional supporter and the love of my life. There is no one I would rather have by my side on this journey.

For my daughters, Arquelle and Sabrina—My miracles, my treasures, and the pride of my life. I love you to the moon and back!

Testimonials

As a Nurse Practitioner Health Coach, I know how vitally important it is to have input from your patients as to how they see themselves becoming well. We as health professionals have a responsibility outside our "Expert" role, and that is as one who encourages the patient to fully engage as an active participant in promoting their own health and well-being. Carole hits this message home as she identifies a 9-Step plan to becoming a Health Champion ... a great read for those who have lost hope in the health system or those embarking on personal wellness goals.

Heather Pitcher, Nurse Practitioner Health Coach, St. John's, Newfoundland and Labrador

My goal as a nurse practitioner is always to empower patients to take control of their own health. Ms. Staveley's book is an excellent tool to help people learn to do exactly that.

Christine McDowell, CD, PHCNP, Ottawa, Ontario

This is such an inspiring and helpful read for anyone facing health challenges. I love how Carole has included the importance of nutrition! Through the use of her own experience she makes a very compelling case for the elimination of inflammatory foods to assist in optimising health. Her forthright honesty is refreshing, especially since she holds no punches by suggesting that the medical professionals do not necessarily have all the answers to an individual's health problems. Carole's own story clearly highlights there is no need to be afraid to question the medical system, especially when you are aiming to find a solution to health challenges.

There are so many useful tips in this book for managing pain. If one approach doesn't work for the reader, she provides a number of options and often rephrases or suggests viewing a problem from a different perspective. Carole has found a way to expertly get inside the reader's head and gives real, effective options—and effectively combats any possible excuses a reader might be clinging on to.
Mandy Mercuri, Self-Pain Management Consultant and Director of Take Hold of Pain, Melbourne, Australia

Having personally suffered with myofascial pain and skeletal issues for decades, I can attest to the challenges and limitations within our current allopathic-based medical system and the mind-shift needed to take personal responsibility for your own health challenges. Once I included holistic nutrition in my life, my healing journey to a pain-free life truly began. Conquer Your Pain in 9 Steps *is not only a fantastic how-to guide on attaining one's health goals, but a heart-warming read of Carole's perseverance and remarkable achievements that will inspire any reader struggling with disease and pain.*
Melody L. Byblow, Registered Holistic Nutritionist, Toronto, Ontario

Acknowledgements

To Those Who Made My Health Champion Journey Possible

Jillian Halligan, M.Sc., B.Sc., C.E.P., my strength coach and friend: For giving me back my life. Thank you for your deep knowledge, your passion for helping others, and your superior problem-solving skills.

Dr. Anthony Galea: For your competence and dedication to the field of sports medicine, and for establishing a multidisciplinary clinic filled with problem solvers determined to help those of us struggling with musculoskeletal conditions.

Dr. Carm Stillo, sports chiropractor: For your effective treatments, your competence, and your unending support as I continued to reach for one impossible goal after another!

My friend MT: For being there when I've needed you most, for your continued support, and for helping me think outside the box to begin solving the mystery of my myofascial dysfunction.

Barrie Shepley, C3 (Canadian Cross Training Club) Head Coach: For creating an environment that encourages triathletes of all levels to train alongside some of the best athletes in the country. And for making us all feel like we belong, no matter how slow we might be.

Dr. William Schoolcraft: For your brilliance and leadership in the field of infertility. You provided the spark that ignited my Health Champion engine. After the birth of my daughters, I recognized the importance of identifying the right health professionals to add to my health team, no matter what health challenge I face.

To Those Who Made This Book Possible

Gina Blakeslee, my coach and mentor: Not only are you an inspiration as a Health Champion and survivor, but your uncanny ability to bring out the best in me has enabled me to push through the challenge of writing this book at a time when I questioned whether I had it in me.

Tina Iaquinta of Modern Concierge: Your reliability and dedication have given me the gift of time, allowing me to focus on the important task of writing and sharing my message.

Julie Salisbury of Influence Publishing: Your passion for getting behind authors who want to make a difference is exemplary. Thank you for your insight on presenting my thoughts to effectively reach the audience that needs to hear my message.

My supportive family: Thank you for being there through thick and thin.

Contents

Prologue: The Story Behind This Book 1

Section I: Establish a Health Champion Mindset 13
    Chapter One: Step 1: Identify What's Holding You Back.................................15
    Chapter Two: Step 2: Establish Your WHY 27
    Chapter Three: Step 3: Set Appropriate Goals 39
    Section I—Summary...50

Section II: Build and Leverage Your Health Champion Team 53
    Chapter Four: Step 4: Develop and Use Your Social Support Network........63
    Chapter Five: Step 5: Select and Challenge the Right Health Professionals.................73
    Chapter Six: Step 6: Budget for Your Healthcare 109
    Section II—Summary..116

Section III: Persevere 119
    Chapter Seven: Step 7: Fully Implement Potential Solutions 121
    Chapter Eight: Step 8: Find Everyday Motivators to Keep You Going........127
    Chapter Nine: Step 9: Never, Ever Give Up! 131
    Section III—Summary..145

Section IV: On Chronic Pain and Triathlons 147
    Chapter Ten: How I Overcame Chronic Myofascial Pain Syndrome...........149
    Chapter Eleven: Triathlon—The Perfect Vehicle for My Health Recovery Journey ..167

Conclusion...193

References and Resources 195
Author Biography...202
About the Author 203

If It's to Be, It's up to Me.
William Johnsen

Prologue—The Story Behind This Book

Compassion is the wish to see others free from suffering.
The Dalai Lama XIV

I am certain that if you're suffering from pain right now, it is possible for you to experience a much healthier, more satisfying life by implementing the steps to becoming your own Health Champion found in this book. I wrote it (as well as my first book, *Not Lying Down*) because I cannot stand the thought of others suffering through years of mental, emotional, or physical pain and living life sub-optimally as I did for years, when there could very well exist solutions to help them conquer or minimize the impact of their pain. And for those of you who simply want to ensure that your future doesn't involve unnecessary suffering, I know this book will help you. Set yourself up as a Health Champion, and you'll be able to deal effectively and efficiently with the health challenges that life will inevitably send your way.

The 9-Step Health Champion approach will help you achieve your full potential by taking you through the entire process, from visualizing your purpose—your reason to persevere—to building the team that will help you address your health challenges most effectively, to maximizing your odds of persevering through it all.

The struggles and triumphs of my Health Champion journey began in the summer of 1996, when I was thirty. I slipped on a wet tennis court and tore a hip muscle, which caused an underlying soft tissue disorder to surface. As I would later discover, this underlying issue led to a chronic myofascial pain syndrome, in which the muscle and fascia (connective tissue found all over our bodies, covering all internal organs) lack the biochemical components to function properly: to stretch, bend, and provide the strength to move at will without injury. This condition also fits the description of fibromyalgia, a diagnosis that seems to be more and more commonly handed out by physicians without much guidance on how to conquer or manage it.

In a matter of months, the hip and back pain that kept me from getting back on the tennis court was the least of my worries. It felt like someone had replaced my muscles and ligaments with metal rods throughout my entire body. It was a struggle to sit, stand, or lie down for any period of time. I was chronically stiff, sore, and uncomfortable. Thus began my search for help within the medical system. Visit after visit to doctors' offices, laboratory and diagnostic facilities, and physiotherapists barely made a dent in my pain and discomfort. Getting to sleep was so difficult. I became chronically tired as a result of the daily battle with pain and the lack of sleep.

After almost a year of complete despair, I eventually learned to push through the pain and adapt my activity level to what my body could tolerate. This meant remaining as active as I could be at the cost of incurring soft tissue injuries at regular intervals. I got back on the tennis court in 1997, but never again reached the level of play I had been accustomed to previously. Between 1996 and 2009, there were many extended breaks from tennis and other activities I enjoyed, because of the chronic pain and stiffness as well as the slew of injuries to which my stiff body was so prone. I spent many hours stretching, rolling on a tennis ball, and taking hot baths in an attempt to relieve the agonizing stiffness that plagued me, so that I could remain somewhat active. There were periods of depression and trying to numb the pain and stiffness with alcohol. I could not understand why the medical community couldn't help me. Having a science background and working in the pharmaceutical industry myself, I was a firm believer in the miracles of mainstream medicine. Where was *my* cure, *my* miracle?

At some level, I began to accept my fate as that of someone who not only would never live out her athletic potential, but who was doomed to a life of pain, frustration, and debilitation. Living an active, athletic life had always been a part of my core being. I felt a rush of exhilaration every time I exerted myself in an effort to improve my athletic skills and fitness level. Having had parents who didn't believe in watching television, I became a fan of athletic activities from a very young age. My older brother is a remarkable athlete and role model—he was captain of his junior hockey teams and gold medalist at the Canadian National Rowing Championships, among other accomplishments. By the time I turned eighteen I had become a self-proclaimed running, fitness, and tennis fanatic. I met my husband during varsity tennis tryouts, and our early married life involved at least two hours of physical fitness or playing tennis every day. I was a bit lost without this level of activity in my life. When I was finally blessed with motherhood, it was heart-wrenching telling my young children that I couldn't carry them, run with them, or even hold up a story book to read to them while lying in bed. After years of being stiff and underutilized, my muscles had also become weak. I had gone from competitive tennis player and avid runner to weak and fragile victim.

The costs of misguided expectations about how to address my chronic pain condition were substantial: thirteen years of pain and stiffness, the loss of athletic undertakings that I cherished, and limited physical engagement in my children's early years. What's even worse, all of it was unnecessary! The resources and solutions were out there, but I misunderstood my role and the role of the medical system in addressing my health problem.

Although I wasn't aware of it yet, my Health Champion

approach began to take shape in 2001 as I battled infertility. With the help of my social network, I uncovered fascinating insights about the vast gaps in competence between infertility "experts." I discovered a clinic with pregnancy rates more than double the national average. Combined with questions borne out of curiosity on my part, this led to the diagnosis and treatment that allowed me to become pregnant with my two beautiful children. I'm certain that this experience strongly influenced my approach to handling my medical issues going forward. Never again would I assume that medical credentials equalled effective problem-solving abilities.

In 2009, when I met an exercise physiologist who explained that my chronic pain condition was likely related to a biochemical issue and could probably be improved through a combination of approaches, I was ready to listen and take action. What she said made total sense, and I was prepared to hunt down every piece of the puzzle to solve my problem. Together with the help of several other health professionals, each with their own expertise (nutrition, chiropractic, sports medicine), we uncovered clues to the underlying problem and put together the suite of approaches to improve my symptoms and ultimately the quality of my life. With the right direction and a lot of hard work, my life completely turned around.

The day I carried my forty-pound daughter up the stairs, I felt I had arrived. After all, what led me to the exercise physiologist in the first place was the desire to get stronger in spite of the pain, so that I could carry my kids and be more active with them. One success led to another. With each month of implementing my nutrition plan, strength workouts, chiropractic treatments, and other modalities uncovered through my new Health Champion lens, I felt I could accomplish more and more. I began training for my first short triathlon and, by the end of 2012, I began to believe I could attempt a full distance triathlon: an IRONMAN event.

It's been a long journey, but I recognize that I'm one of the lucky ones. I figured it out. I can now live my life on my own terms and I'm not looking back on what might have been. Those thirteen years of suffering have given me an immense gift—the gift of becoming a Health Champion—which I am compelled to share with the world. I simply could not stand by and let this happen to others. This book is a product of my mission to share my gift.

Please note that I'm not promising cures or miracles. The objective of this book is to empower you to reach your fullest potential by helping you take control of your health challenges and become your own Health Champion. The 9 Steps I present are drawn from my lessons learned in conquering thirteen years of debilitating chronic pain. The fact that I was able to train for and complete an IRONMAN triathlon just four short years after discovering the winning approach to dealing with my condition indicated to me that much of my suffering had been unnecessary; that there had been solutions out there all along. But why wasn't I offered these solutions in the hundreds of medical visits I attended?

The answer lies in the concept of ownership of one's health—what I call being your own Health Champion. Although I was booking appointments and showing up for them, I didn't understand that I needed to be the one owning the responsibility for solving the problem.

What I hope you will take away from this book, first and foremost, is that you are ultimately in charge of defining and achieving your healthiest state of being. Many of you will nod your heads in agreement, but are you truly embracing the responsibility for solving your health challenges, whatever they may be? When you walk into a doctor's office, do you approach the interaction from the point of view of a team leader, a Chief Problem Solver consulting with one of many resources in your health network? Do you regularly challenge health professionals to provide more details, greater insights, additional resources, or input on what actions you can take to speed up the recovery process? Do you approach health appointments prepared to discuss a hypothesis about your condition?

The 9-Step Health Champion approach presented in this book is underpinned by the three following principles:

1. It is critical to establish a purposeful and problem-solving mindset related to your health.
2. You must build and leverage a team of knowledgeable, supportive, and resourceful people to assist you in your quest to fulfill your healthiest potential.
3. You must expect that perseverance will be required on your journey. To that end, you need tools, resources, and relationships that inspire and motivate you to keep moving forward.

As grateful as I am for having discovered the approach and solutions to help me effectively manage my condition, I don't want anyone else to suffer longer than necessary. I am 99 percent certain that whatever your current health problem is, you can obtain better care, regain hope for a better future, and get more out of life than you believe possible. It starts with taking control of your healthcare, becoming informed about your condition, following clear guidelines to search for the right health professionals, asking a lot of questions, and never, ever giving up. While it took me thirteen years of trial and error and another four years of further methodical searching to gather all the information I needed to fulfill my potential, I truly hope you can apply my insights to your current situation and reach a better health state much sooner. The goal is to suffer less and achieve more.

By "achieving more," I don't mean you have to train for an IRONMAN triathlon! But if I was able to achieve that (3.8 km swim, 180 km bike, 42.2 km run) after starting out with a goal of running just a couple of kilometers without injury, there are possibilities awaiting you that you haven't even dreamt of yet. And the rewards—well, the rewards are difficult to put into words. But the thoughts that came into my mind on that beautiful day in 2013, as I entered the water to begin my 226 km (140.6 mile) IRONMAN journey might help describe the feeling. My thoughts were, "I am so fortunate. I am free. I want others to feel this. I don't want anyone suffering more than they need to." There was a sense of total liberation inside me. I had found my new purpose in life.

Taking on the Health Champion mindset and approach will likely require you to make some behavioral changes. But behavioral change is not easy, and thirty years of research document the fact that a specific change process must be followed in order to achieve lasting success (John Norcross, *Changeology*, Simon & Schuster, 2012). The steps outlined in this book are ordered in such a way as to facilitate the process of morphing yourself into a Health Champion for the long term. The 9 Steps are broken down into three sections, each building on the previous one.

Section I—Establish a Health Champion Mindset—focuses on getting yourself psyched and prepared for your journey. It will help you set yourself up for success and set appropriate goals before jumping into action.

Section II—Build and Leverage Your Health Champion Team—this is the "action" stage, focused on how to identify individuals (both inside and outside the healthcare system) who are most likely to help you resolve your health challenges, and how to best leverage all the health resources that can start you on the road to suffering less, achieving more, and fulfilling your life purpose.

Section III—Persevere—is all about following through in the short and long term, and fully internalizing the Health

Champion approach so as to minimize your suffering time and maximize your achievements.

At the end of each of the three sections, I offer a summary that includes a checklist to help you recognize whether or not you're ready to move on to the next section, or if you need to spend a bit more time reviewing and implementing the steps presented in the section. Jumping too quickly from one section to the next can reduce your chances of achieving lasting success as a Health Champion.

In Chapters 1 to 9, which deal with becoming a Health Champion, I provide some thought-provoking questions and exercises. Taking the time to ponder the questions and working through the exercises will allow you to maximize the benefits you will receive from reading this book. My job is to help raise your awareness and to provide some inspiration and guidance based on my own experiences and discoveries. The choice to implement the information and become your own Health Champion is completely in your hands.

Section IV—On Chronic Pain and Triathlons—addresses my personal journey in more detail. Chapter 10 provides some background on chronic myofascial pain syndrome, its impact on my life, and the multiple approaches I uncovered to improve my condition. Chapter 11 covers how I embraced triathlon as the vehicle for measuring improvements in my physical health and for keeping me challenged to find new approaches to enhance my health. I provide some tips on getting started with triathlon in case my story inspires you to give the sport a try as a motivational driver and a yardstick for improvement as you progress on your Health Champion journey.

It's Time for a Health Champion Revolution

The tendency in Western societies is to bring our problems to a medical practitioner, and then "hand it over," expecting the expert to solve it. There are three primary characteristics of North American healthcare models that tend to drive this expectation:

1. A third party is often paying, sending the message that someone else knows who and what is best to address our health concerns ("If it's 'covered,' it's good medicine.").
2. The model is based on "patching up" health breakdowns versus achieving the optimal health outcome for each individual.
3. Since physicians are trained to fix many health problems, they are often regarded as the authorities on all health-related issues. However, it is well established that the majority are not adequately trained in many aspects of achieving and maintaining optimal health. This is particularly the case when it comes to the diagnosis and management of conditions like chronic pain.

Dr. Manon Bolliger, in her book *What Patients Don't Say if Doctors Don't Ask*, conveys to physicians the importance of the patient's involvement and the doctor-patient relationship in the healing process. She addresses the fact that the pain a patient feels will often not match any "objective" tests conducted by the physician. Doctor and patient must both be committed to addressing the problem in order for healing to take place. The patient's role is at least as important as that of the physician. Every individual presents with a background that differs in genetics, upbringing, traumatic experiences, and the ability to tolerate stress and pain, among many other aspects. "Treating a 'disease' without treating the person who developed it is pointless," according to Dr. Bolliger.

Just as doctors can influence patients, the inverse is true.[1] Patient characteristics and behaviors can influence the way a physician practices.[2] As Chief Problem Solvers on our health journey, we must not look to medical professionals as our problem solvers. Rather, let's be the problem solvers seeking input from a variety of health resources, including medical professionals. Although this sounds like a minor shift, it is in fact a monumental one. If we wholeheartedly implement this approach, I'm convinced we can revolutionize the healthcare system and achieve better health outcomes with a more efficient use of health resources.

Let's stop believing that medical professionals hold the keys to our health breakthroughs. We have so much more power to determine our health outcomes than we realize. It's a matter of taking ownership and applying a consumer-like mindset to the task of uncovering the approaches to our healthiest potential.

I want to emphasize the potentially life-changing role that a good problem solver can have within the healthcare system. Whether he is a GP, a nurse, a physiotherapist, a nutritionist, or a naturopath, the health professional MUST look at the individual's health problem in a holistic, multidisciplinary way. By "holistic," I mean looking more deeply into what the source of the problem might be, taking into account nutrition, exercise, and other lifestyle habits. A holistic approach also involves looking beyond what conventional Western medicine has to offer, recognizing that many alternative approaches can bring much relief for many conditions. And health professionals must involve the patient as a problem-solving partner in the process.

One of the frustrations I have with physicians is that many of them are trained to ignore anything outside the traditional

---

[1]planetreegrove.com/wp-content/uploads/2013/05/Mutual-influence-in-shared-decision-making.pdf

[2]adc.bmj.com/content/84/6/459.full; and ncbi.nlm.nih.gov/pubmed/7109746

medical system. What they usually offer are medications and surgery, with physiotherapist or nutritionist referrals at the outer limits. I had a chronic pain problem that didn't fit within the scope of practice of Western medicine. No clear diagnosis was established through "objective" testing. The winning solution to my pain was an integrated, holistic approach that crossed over disciplines such as nutrition, chiropractic, physical therapy, and exercise physiology—combined with a lot of effort on my part. Not one doctor among the dozens I met in thirteen years indicated that I might benefit from a combination of non-medical and medical interventions. There is a massive gap between how physicians are trained and the holistic approach required to ensure many individuals obtain optimal care based on their particular health problem and individual characteristics. This issue is magnified in chronic conditions, whether or not a clear diagnosis is established.

I was glad to see chronic pain addressed in the news recently on the CBC, Canada's national news network.[3] In one article, there was an acknowledgement from physicians in British Columbia that not enough time is spent on pain management in medical training. Dr. Michael Negraeff, one of the physicians spearheading a chronic pain training program for family doctors, states that "chronic pain is really an orphaned condition in medicine." In fact, Canadian veterinary students receive five times more training in pain management than Canadian medical students.

These disturbing facts about Western medicine played a large role in my thirteen-year trial-and-error search for the answers to my chronic myofascial pain syndrome. After finally stumbling across the answers, I felt the need to convert my search process into a systematic approach to help others find solutions to their health challenges sooner rather than later. Whether

---

[3] cbc.ca/news/canada/british-columbia/chronic-pain-training-introduced-for-b-c-s-family-doctors-1.2626294

you're frustrated with the medical establishment or simply looking for ways to improve your health status to get more out of life, please give my Health Champion approach a try. What do you have to lose?

The Vision for an Empowered and Healthier Future

My mission extends beyond helping individuals become Health Champions. The long-term vision is to contribute to the development of a society filled with Health Champions. Within such a society, health professionals will have no choice but to embrace the fact that the individual must be the leader of the health team working to solve his or her health challenge. Once this mind-shift occurs, the overall health and quality of life of our population will improve. More individuals will be empowered to strive for and achieve their full potential, leading to a healthier, more productive, and more satisfied society. Not to mention the fact that an empowered population will put much less strain on the healthcare system, giving us the much-needed breathing room to implement the reforms that governments and employers have been preaching for years. This broad-scale impact begins with each one of us and our individual Health Champion journeys.

Confucius said, "To put the world right in order, we must first put the nation in order; to put the nation in order, we must first put the family in order; to put the family in order, we must first cultivate our personal life; we must first set our hearts right."

Our current approach to healthcare (both from an individual and systems perspective) is unsustainable. It is time for a Health Champion revolution! I invite you to join me in fulfilling this critical mission.

SECTION I

Establish a Health Champion Mindset

The Health Champion mindset is essentially about setting yourself up to become your own Chief Problem Solver when it comes to health matters. You need to believe that improvements are possible, and that you have the power to discover and implement the tools and approaches that will get you there. By first understanding the beliefs and behaviors that are keeping you in your current state of health, then establishing a purpose that will drive you forward, and setting appropriate goals, you will be in the right state of mind to take action on your Health Champion journey.

Each of the three chapters in this section include questions and exercises that can really help you get into the right mindset. Chapter 2, Step 2: Establish Your WHY, includes exercises that might require you to spend several hours thinking about your life purpose and how you can use it to propel yourself forward. Please don't rush through these exercises as they are pivotal to your ultimate success in implementing the 9 Steps and achieving your healthiest potential.

What will it mean for you to get healthier and feel better? What will be the impact on your life and on the lives of others around you? What first step can you take on your health improvement journey? Let's begin building that mindset.

One

Step 1: Identify What's Holding You Back

When we focus on numbing the pain, we stifle our greatest opportunities for growth.

In addition to the health concern(s) that might be keeping you from living your life on your own terms, we need to explore what underlying thought processes, beliefs, and expectations might be at play in keeping you from advancing on your journey toward a healthier you. Can you say with confidence that you've taken all the steps necessary to improve your current health condition? If not, why not?

Looking back on my own journey, one of the most significant obstacles that got in the way of reclaiming my active life was the belief that the medical system held the "magic bullet" cure for my condition. Although I couldn't articulate it, this belief was something that was carved deeply into my subconscious, fed by the cultural norms and expectations ingrained in me from a young age. The unconscious message goes something like, "If something in your body isn't functioning properly, it's a doctor's job to figure out why and to fix it." This was such an unquestioned belief, that it wasn't possible for me to identify it and realize that it might be an obstacle to my progress. In my mind, I was "taking charge of my health" by booking and attending medical appointments. Surely one of these doctors would tell me what was wrong and send me home with the elixir that would cure me.

The following example illustrates how such a deeply buried belief can hinder your progress. In the first few years of my struggles with pain, I experienced a few physical therapy techniques that seemed to provide some partial relief, but for some reason I didn't pursue them with any energy. I was still focused on the negative impact of my condition and subconsciously looking for the big bang of success that would come from an external force—something that would be done *to* me like a procedure or a prescription I would take. I felt that when I found "the answer" I would know it, and all the pain and stiffness would subside permanently. Until then, I was resigned to a less-than-optimal life. I felt helpless. As I mentioned in the Prologue, I turned to alcohol as a way to numb the pain and discomfort, and sank into a depressed state. I realize now that my efforts to numb the pain only kept me focused on the negative, on my existing situation. Further, they reduced my ability to envision what was possible and to look for solutions.

Seeing the Forest Versus the Trees

In thinking about your current health challenge, how much of your focus is on the problem itself and what it is keeping you from doing? Are you focused on "taking the edge off" and minimizing the suffering? By contrast, how much of your focus is on reaching your healthiest state, despite this health challenge? What about all the possible approaches out there that might help you conquer or manage your condition, just waiting for you to uncover them? What does your gut tell you about additional diagnostics or solutions that you haven't yet uncovered? Even with a firm diagnosis, are you certain you've explored all the options that will allow you to function at the highest level possible?

I understand that in many cases, there needs to be some pain management in order to enable you to function at a minimum level. This is an important step and one you clearly need to work on with your doctor or other health professional(s). The problem comes when we start to look at pain reduction (usually with prescription drugs or self-administered pain-numbing substances) as the long-term solution. I urge you to consider the fact that pain reduction or pain management is only the first step on your journey! Look at pain as an *enabler* that allows you to begin your journey to a healthier state.

This chapter lays the groundwork for you to think in terms of the "forest"—the whole picture that puts your health challenge in perspective and allows you to examine the thought processes that might be serving to keep you stuck in your current situation. Esteemed economist John Maynard Keynes once wrote "the difficulty lies not so much in developing new ideas as in escaping from old ones." This is about opening your mind to new ways of thinking that could shatter your current beliefs about your long-term health prospects.

Before you begin listing all the external factors (outside your control) keeping you from progressing to the next level of wellness, it's important to take some time and examine your own internal factors—the things you can control. An important concept to consider at this stage is mindfulness or self-awareness. I like to think of this as spying on our own thought processes. Before you can have a meaningful conversation about the thought processes, beliefs, or expectations that are holding you back, you need to be able to practice at least some basic level of mindfulness, which means observing those thought processes in action. The challenge here is that we're often trying to observe thoughts that have been buried for years, filed in the brain's archives as "accepted fact" and no longer recognized as active thought processes. As mentioned earlier, my beliefs that the only place to look for answers to my chronic pain was in the medical system and that I was not responsible for finding solutions didn't even occur to me as being thought processes until I received a "wake-up call."

There is often so much information flying through our brains that it's easy to forget that our thought process is ultimately within our control. Knowing we can take control, however, doesn't mean it's easy to do so. Deeply rooted, subconscious beliefs including those pertaining to our self-worth are often at play without our knowledge, sabotaging our ability to take on the behaviors we know are necessary to improve our current situation. In my thirties I came to the realization that self-worth is at the heart of so many human behaviors, particularly those behaviors affecting our health and wellness. If you don't value yourself, then why would you take on behaviors that are good for your health and self-esteem?

If self-worth is an issue for you, the hardest part is figuring out why you don't value yourself. Once you've identified the reason behind that, getting past it becomes realistic because of your greater awareness. If you can do some soul-searching and at least identify what circumstances in your past could have led you to have low self-worth, then that is a step toward being able to overcome this sentiment. I am not a psychologist, so I am simply stating my observations over a lifetime of discovering my own self-worth.

I recently viewed a TED Talk by Brené Brown, a Ph.D. Social Science Research Professor at the University of Houston and author.[4] She really struck a chord with me on the self-destructive behaviors displayed by many in our society. Essentially, she is saying that those who live "wholeheartedly" believe they are worthy of love and belonging. This "wholehearted" cohort has the following characteristics:

1. *Courage*: the ability to embrace being imperfect;
2. *Compassion*: the ability to be kind to themselves so that they can feel compassion for others;
3. *Vulnerability*: the belief that what makes them vulnerable also makes them beautiful.

---

[4]ted.com/talks/brene_brown_on_vulnerability.html

Many of us fear vulnerability and liken it to weakness. We try to numb it; we deny our responsibility in wrongdoings; we try to perfect the world around us. If we can embrace vulnerability and believe that we are truly "enough" as we are, we would be so much kinder to ourselves and to others. My point is that every one of us is worthy of doing all that we can to be the healthiest, strongest, and fittest person we can be while accepting and appreciating ourselves at every stage in the process. I highly recommend watching Brené's twenty-minute TED talk on vulnerability.

As part of the process of introspection to identify and understand what could be holding you back, try answering the following questions as honestly as you can:

- How do you handle adversity?

    Do you feel defeated the moment something goes wrong, or do you welcome adversity as an opportunity to propel yourself to greater heights?

- Do you accept and value yourself for who you are, or do you have a deep underlying belief that you're not worthy?

    Although this feeling is often difficult to pinpoint due to its frequently subconscious nature, you can get around it by focusing on others instead of yourself. Can you think about the contributions you could make in others' lives if you were healthier? Have you given much thought to your strengths rather than to your limitations?

- Are you trying to numb the negative emotions linked to your health problems, or are you facing them head-on?

    Psychologist Steven Hayes, Ph.D. articulates it well. He says that in order to minimize the impact of negative thoughts and emotions, we must first "be with them" and acknowledge them. My key takeaways from a talk he recently gave were that "Pain is a necessary part of life, and can be life-enhancing" and "Love and loss come as an Oreo cookie—you can't separate them!"[5] My Health Champion interpretation of these insights is as follows: Whatever the problem holding you back (mental, emotional, or physical), it is necessary to delve into the pain before you can get past it.

If the thoughts I've shared so far in this chapter are causing you to feel anxious or distressed, or if you believe there is a need to delve into your past in order to address some of the suppressed negative emotions that might be causing you to sabotage your own well-being, I encourage you to seek the help of a psychiatrist or a qualified therapist or counselor. Begin by seeking a recommendation from a trusted health professional.

Practicing Gratitude

Gratitude is an important habit to cultivate in order to foster a psychological environment that supports self-worth and sets the stage for becoming a Health Champion. You might be wondering why I describe gratitude as a habit. After reading Dr. Brené Brown's book, *The Gifts of Imperfection*, I realized the importance of consciously practicing gratitude; of taking the time to mindfully recognize all the things in my life for which I should be grateful.

On my birthday last year, I reflected on why I should be grateful for turning forty-eight. As far as self-worth and personal satisfaction are concerned, I can honestly say that I don't miss my twenties and thirties. I feel so fortunate and grateful for so many things that have really come to fruition in this fifth decade of my life, including the following:

---

[5]See Dr. Hayes' website: stevenchayes.com

1. understanding the importance of seeking my own solutions to health challenges, and achieving a better level of health and fitness than I could ever imagine;
2. having the opportunity to realize an incredible dream of participating in an IRONMAN;
3. receiving the gift of raising my beautiful daughters;
4. having the most supportive husband I could ever ask for (who's still around after twenty-three years!);
5. finding my life's mission of empowering others to conquer health challenges and to reach their physical potential;
6. deepening friendships and new relationships with some amazing people that I admire so much.

I guess there is enough there to offset my only complaint about getting older—the appearance of wrinkles! Adopting a practice of consciously listing those things for which you are grateful can help you get into the right mindset to take on your health challenges. Once you start to focus on the positives in your life, you begin to look for ways to build on those positives, rather than dwelling on the negatives—those things that are holding you back.

What I'm learning is that gratitude is closely linked with joy. Dr. Brené Brown's extensive research has revealed that the opposite of joy is not sadness but rather fear. Fear is often the culprit that holds us back. Whether it is fear of failure or fear of the changes that success might bring, it is important to examine whether or not fear hides behind our inability to set high goals and keep moving forward.

Developing Your Strengths and Viewing Your Weaknesses as Opportunities

I thought the following two stories, taken from separate TED talks, might inspire you to focus on moving forward and setting your sights on what's possible.

Baby Mario Overcomes a Severe Stroke

A ten-day old child suffered a stroke that wiped out the right side of his brain. The prognosis from doctors was that he would never be able to use the left side of his body. After months of focusing on "the problem," his parents realized that their baby would never reach his full potential unless they helped him develop his strengths.

For the next two and a half years, Mario's parents acted as mirrors and showed him the full potential of what he could accomplish. Through this practice, Mario's brain was conditioned to believe he was fully functional. Mario is now walking unassisted.

The key message in this story, relayed in a short and inspiring TED Talk video, is to focus on what you can become, not on the problems that are holding you back.[6]

Amy Purdy Soars Beyond Her Physical Limitations

My corporate experience taught me that the more limited your budget, the more creative you need to be with your marketing resources. Why shouldn't we look at our limitations in the same light? Every limitation is an opportunity to get creative, and still accomplish what we want in life—in a new way.

Amy Purdy's ten-minute TED Talk is a powerful example of someone who could have chosen to focus on what her new limitations prevented her from doing.[7] After recovering from bacterial meningitis and the loss of her spleen, kidneys, hearing in one ear, and both legs below the knee, Purdy chose to use her imagination, and visualized how she could still accomplish what she wanted in life in a whole new way, *because* of her limitations.

---

[6] ted.com/talks/roberto_d_angelo_francesca_fedeli_in_our_baby_s_illness_a_life_lesson.html
[7] ted.com/talks/amy_purdy_living_beyond_limits

After several months of mourning the loss of the active twenty-year-old life she knew, Amy asked herself how she could rewrite her life's story. She began to think of what she *could* do, *because* of her new limitations. Not only did she find a prosthetic designer with whom to collaborate in designing the types of legs that would best serve her goals, she used those legs to eventually become a two-time World Cup Champion in adaptive snowboarding. Amy says that borders and obstacles can either stop us in our tracks or force us to become creative. Rather than trying to break down our borders, can we push off them and see how far they might take us?

Now that you've begun to identify and look beyond your limitations, I'd like to take you through a brief exercise that can begin to stretch your imagination and plant the seed of what might be possible.

The Magic Wand Exercise

If I had a magic wand with the power to bestow upon you your ideal state of wellness, what would you ask for? There are no barriers, no limitations. This is magic. You can get exactly what you want, no questions asked. This is something you definitely could not reach tomorrow, and you have no idea how you could get there, but it's really desirable for you. Be as specific as possible—include actions. What would you be *doing*?

Now, considering your ideal situation, what types of things would need to happen in order for you to get there? List five positives in your life that could contribute to getting you closer to that ideal state of wellness you described above. These can be your own strengths, resources available to you, or supportive people who are in your life.

Positives in My Life:

1. ____
2. ____
3. ____
4. ____
5. ____

List five things that you *should* be doing, in order to achieve your healthiest life.

Things I Should Be Doing:

1. ____
2. ____
3. ____
4. ____
5. ____

What expectations and beliefs do you hold that might get in the way of doing what you know you should be doing? For example, expecting that anything less than hundred percent perfect health is not worth pursuing; or believing you've done everything you could; or believing that it's easier for other people.

Expectations/Beliefs That Could Be Getting in My Way:

1. ____
2. ____
3. ____
4. ____
5. ____

Once you recognize and overcome the psychological issues holding you back, you will likely still need to deal with the more conscious thought processes and behaviors that underlie your inability to move forward toward finding solutions and improving your quality of life. Many of these will be addressed in upcoming chapters. The following questions can help you begin the process of identifying whether or not you've truly done everything within your power to get healthier and fulfill your potential:

- Have you identified your greater purpose, your vision of how a healthier you could contribute to making the world a better place? I call this "establishing your WHY."
- Are you setting specific, achievable, and measurable goals for what "progress" looks like for you? Are these goals aligned with your WHY?
- Do you consciously spend more time with people who are positive and supportive, and seek to minimize your time spent with people who bring you down?
- Have you shared your health challenges with your social network, and allowed them to share insights and recommendations with you? If so, have you taken action on these insights and recommendations?
- Have you researched and requested access to the best doctors and health professionals specializing in your particular condition?
- Are you keeping an open mind about the definition of "Health Professional"? How far outside mainstream medicine have you looked for approaches that could complement the mainstream approach?
- Are you leading the discussion every time you see a health professional? Do you attend every appointment prepared to ask questions from research you've done?
- When a health professional disappoints you consistently,

do you just keep going back or worse yet, just give up on getting help?

- Are you budgeting for your healthcare needs? Although many health services could be paid for by a medical plan, there are a multitude of health resources out there that might not be covered, but that could provide some key solutions to your health challenge. Where is the bulk of your disposable income going right now?
- For every recommendation made by a health professional, how well have you followed through to evaluate the usefulness of the recommendation or treatment? Have you fully understood the rationale behind the recommendation or treatment? Do you know how long you need to implement the treatment, exercise regime, nutrition plan, etc., before seeing its full impact?
- Have you developed personal motivation strategies that can help you stay on track, especially on the days when you want to throw in the towel?

I hope the following chapters will give you what you need to transform yourself into a Health Champion, and that you have the opportunity to experience the personal power and satisfaction that comes from being in charge of your own health. Although there will be no "cure" for many of us with chronic conditions, I know from personal experience that the Health Champion approach can lead to a much healthier and more satisfying life journey, despite an underlying condition.

Two

Step 2: Establish Your WHY

*He who has a strong enough WHY can bear
almost any HOW.*
Attributed to Friedrich Nietzsche

Your WHY is what ignites that inner light. The more you focus
on your WHY, the brighter the light will burn.

What I'm trying to get at here is essentially your Life Purpose
statement. I want to help you answer the question: How will
I make the world just a little bit better, in my own way? As
human beings, we have an innate need for community. When
you think about individuals who have left their mark on the
world by making it a better place, the impact has typically been
achieved through sharing their unique gifts with others. In
other words, our Life Purpose is typically defined by sharing
ourselves with others.

*Every individual has a place to fill in the world
and is important in some respect whether he
chooses to be so or not.*
Nathaniel Hawthorne

How Purpose Can Trump Fear

I share the following story to help you recognize just how
powerful a purpose statement can be. It is essentially the light
at the end of the tunnel that can propel you past any fear or
adversity that you might be faced with on your journey.

Many years ago, at the beginning of my career, I took a job

as a Pharmaceutical Sales Representative. The combination of a science degree and an MBA made me a perfect candidate for the pharmaceuticals industry, which I had targeted through my career search.

After acing the four-week training program, I was excited about getting out there and sharing my technical knowledge with doctors. What I discovered on my first day "flying solo" was that I needed to "sell" myself to the receptionists before having a chance to meet with the doctors. Who was I kidding? I wasn't a sales person. I could never be a sales person. It just wasn't me.

Overwhelmed with fear and apprehension about my career choice, I drove straight home, crawled under my bed covers and assumed the fetal position, saying to myself, "What was I thinking? I can't do this. I've made a huge mistake. What am I going to do? I'm not a sales person."

Suddenly, I had a moment of strength and told myself, "You're not in this to be a sales person. You're in this to help doctors provide better care to their patients. You know the data about your products better than anyone else. By helping doctors understand how the appropriate use of these products can help patients get better, you are making a difference in people's lives. Maybe you didn't go to medical school, but this could be your way of contributing to medical care."

As I started to think about this role in terms of my passion for improving people's health, the fear and anxiety subsided. I was able to gather up my courage, get back out there, and approach the medical offices with confidence drawn from my renewed sense of purpose.

Thinking back to my 2013 IRONMAN race, I have to say I was gripped with a similar sense of fear the night before. As I stood looking out at the thousands of bikes set up in the transition area, I felt this sudden sense of panic. I heard a voice in my head saying, "It's okay to back out. No one will hold it against you. You were never expected to get this far."

But I quickly turned my thoughts to how the completion of the IRONMAN would give me the credibility to spread the word about the power of becoming your own Health Champion to overcome health challenges. The IRONMAN would give me the fuel to complete my book and launch my company, Inner Victory Coaching.[8] Once again, purpose trumped fear.

How can you make the connection between your Health Champion journey, your passions, and your purpose?

When I look back to the days when chronic myofascial pain ruled my life, my WHY for pushing through the adversity and searching for solutions became clearer as my desire for playing an active role in my children's lives increased. At that time, my community was my immediate family, my children in particular. I wanted to give of myself to my kids. This was a much more powerful force to propel me forward than a statement like "I want the pain to stop."

Your Life Purpose statement or WHY will likely evolve over time, depending on many factors such as life stage, the desire to have a positive impact on a broader community, a changed perspective based on a life-altering event, etc. Using my example, once I was able to manage my condition and become more physically engaged with my kids, I recognized the opportunity to use my journey as a way to help others overcome their own health challenges. My passion for athletics and for having an impact in the health field drove me to paint a new WHY vision: "To help thousands of others who are suffering needlessly."

Persevering through the training and completion of an IRONMAN triathlon while managing a chronic pain condition was fuelled by my desire to build a powerful message that could impact the lives of many. This new WHY was based on a desire to share myself with others, but this time the community extended well beyond that of my family.

---

[8]carolestaveley.com

Discovering Your WHY

The following are some questions and visualization exercises designed to help you uncover the WHY behind your optimal life. Whether or not you have already given this some thought, the process of going through the exercises can help you further crystallize your WHY. If you're trying to get through this book as quickly as you can, keep in mind, this isn't necessarily something you can complete in one sitting. You will likely need to process these questions and visualizations over several days or even weeks. You might want to make a note in your calendar to come back and think through these exercises daily over the next week or so.

1. How will your life be different when you improve your health and wellness?
   a. Can you list both internal and external factors?
   b. Look at your answers. Have you listed things like the types of behaviors you would be exhibiting, or how you would feel?
   c. As you review each answer, can you ask yourself "why" it would matter that these things will be different in your life? Dig deep. Why would it really matter if all these things were different or better? Whose lives could you impact positively when you achieve a better health state?
2. Think about what you're good at, and what you're passionate about. How could you use these to make the world around you just a little bit better? What kind of difference could you make in the lives of others that would make you feel that your life has been worthwhile?
   a. Thinking about who and what you can impact in the world can be as narrow or broad as you want—immediate family and friends versus a global community or a system that impacts a community.
   b. What is your "gift" to the world?

By this point, you might have "seen the light." Maybe you now know your purpose, your WHY, and you've been filled with powerful emotion when thinking about realizing this purpose of yours. You now know that your WHY will carry you through all the difficulties, the setbacks, the adversities related to achieving that optimal state you'd like to find yourself in.

Then again, maybe you're not there yet. The following are two visualization exercises that might help you free up your mind in order to access some powerful insights that are buried deep in your subconscious. You can choose to do one or both of these, depending on how close you are to articulating your WHY at this point.

Begin by sitting as comfortably as possible. Take five deep breaths through the nose, and exhale through the mouth. Make the inhales and exhales last as long as possible. Try to relax every part of your body to the point where you feel like someone could come along and knock you off your chair without much effort.

Visualization A

Go back to a time in your life when you felt your full power. Your whole body tingled with excitement and you simply didn't care what anyone thought of you. You were absolutely alive and at peace with yourself. Now answer the following:

- Where were you?
- What were you doing?
- Who was around you?
- What impact were you having on them?
- How were they behaving?

Visualization B

You are getting into a spacecraft. The spacecraft takes off. You are on your way to an undeveloped planet in the universe. It's a fine planet in every way, but it's uninhabited. You have the power to create any type of environment you want on this planet. It can be any way you want it to be, populated with anyone you want. You get to make up all the rules and guidelines. When you land, what will you make happen? What is the impact you want to have that will make this planet the way you want it to be?

Take a moment to think about it, then describe the way you want your planet to be. In particular, focus on the impact you personally will have on making this happen.

From the above exercises, can you begin to formulate something that resembles a "life purpose statement" or a WHY? A higher purpose that will give you great satisfaction to fulfill? A unique difference you can make in the world—whether in your immediate social circle or beyond?

Can you see how taking action toward your healthiest or optimal state can help you fulfill your purpose? Keep your WHY at the front of your mind's eye all the time. It will pull you through some of your most challenging times. And if you don't think you've found your WHY just yet, don't worry. It's not always obvious. You've made progress simply by doing these exercises. Go back through the information and keep asking yourself WHY any of this stuff would matter. What will make it all meaningful? What is it that would make you feel like you've fully shared your gifts with the world?

I've talked about an evolution in your WHY; the fact that your purpose can evolve over time. As you progress forward and begin to fulfill what you initially set out as your purpose, you need to keep revisiting the concept of WHY. According to Simon Sinek, author of *Start With Why*, our deepest underlying purpose or WHY actually never changes.[9] The problem is

---

[9] *Start with Why: How Great Leaders Inspire Everyone to Take Action*, Penguin Group, 2009

that it's difficult to articulate. Once you have a taste of living your life in alignment with your true purpose, you'll feel it. You'll begin to unveil that deepest purpose that's lying dormant within you, and it will become easier to articulate.

My approach to dealing with the fact that your ultimate WHY can be difficult to articulate is to find a WHY that you *can* articulate right now, something that's as deep in your unconscious as you can reach today, then allow it to evolve over time. You'll know when you're heading in the right direction, because when you're fulfilling your purpose, your passion is ignited. Eventually your true, unchanging WHY will reveal itself.

To arrive at your true WHY, you need to keep asking yourself "Why?" many times. Your first answer is almost guaranteed not to be the true WHY. Below is an example of what a typical answer might be to the question, "Why do you want to be as healthy as you can be?" It is followed by a line of questioning that could get you closer to a deeper answer that could drive a change in your behavior:

- **Question**: "Why do you want to be as healthy as you can be?"
- **First Answer**: "Because I want to feel better."
- **Next Question**: "Why do you want to feel better?"
- **Answer**: "So I can be less tired and frustrated at the end of the day."
- **Next Question**: "Why do you want to be less tired and frustrated at the end of the day?"
- **Answer**: "So I can spend quality time with my kids."
- **Next Question**: "Why do you want to spend quality time with your kids?"
- **Answer**: "Because I want them to know how much I love them."
- **Next Question**: "And why will it make a difference if they know you love them?"

- **Answer**: "It will make a difference because when kids feel loved, they are more likely to become positive people who can make a difference in the world."

Now we're getting closer to the WHY! Of course, this is just an example and everyone's WHY will be different. But hopefully you get the idea and the importance of really digging deep to uncover the WHY for you to begin the journey to your healthiest possible state, no matter what your starting point is.

The above example of arriving at a WHY statement is close to what was going through my mind as a new mother still struggling with chronic pain. As I began to feel better, my WHY evolved into empowering others to improve their lives through sharing my story. I recently went through the exercise again, trying to articulate my deepest, unchanging purpose, and I came up with two words: *maximizing potential*. When I look back to the "Whys" that drove me this far (for example, engaging with my kids and enabling others to fulfill their potential), these were directly in line with this overall, deep-rooted purpose of maximizing potential. Now that I'm able to articulate it, I don't need to go any further to establish my WHY. Everything I do in life is guided by maximizing potential—mine, my children's, my clients', and anyone else's who will listen to my message. When I stray from this purpose, I quickly become aware of a dip in my passion and motivation, and know that it's time to reconnect with my WHY.

An interesting fact emerged from research on the aging process. A purpose-driven life is a higher quality life, and is likely tied to greater longevity (Bruce Grierson).[10] In other words, whether establishing your WHY leads you directly to solving your health condition or not, living with purpose will give you

---

[10]*What Makes Olga Run*, Random House Canada, 2014

a better life experience. We all need to feel that we matter and that we can make a difference.

Find your purpose, and you will likely find yourself:

- happier;
- more apt to set challenging goals;
- more able to persevere through the difficult times.

One of the most powerful reminders of this can be found in holocaust survivor Viktor E. Frankl's book, *Man's Search For Meaning.*[11] Stripped of all possessions and having lost almost all of his loved ones during his horrific concentration camp experience, Frankl reflected on the human psyche's ability to pursue life in the face of such hopeless circumstances. He concluded that finding one's true meaning in life, often by overcoming tragedy, is the way to achieve a deep sense of personal satisfaction and ultimately to contribute to improving the state of our world. There are multiple sources of social and psychological research pointing toward the fact that happiness and motivation are closely tied to having a sense of purpose.

What Does It Mean to Be as Healthy as You Can Be?

As I mentioned earlier, my goal is not to cure you of your ailments, but rather to help you reach your healthiest state so that you can suffer less and ultimately accomplish more in your life. Many of us have chronic health conditions that probably won't go away; however, we often don't recognize the opportunity presented to us through the adversity. If we allow ourselves to focus on how far we can go instead of on our limitations, our lives will improve regardless of the state of our underlying health condition. And the upside of taking this approach is the motivation to continue pursuing new approaches to better health.

---

[11]Washington Square Press, 1984

Though I now consider myself "as healthy as I can be," I realize that this is a continuous improvement process, a state of mind. Does it mean no pain, or a high-performance body that never breaks down? Not at all, as my myofascial disorder still exists. What it does mean is that I can see a path to continuous improvements in my physical functioning, I have the confidence to overcome setbacks, and I can dare to set more and more challenging goals for myself (like completing an IRONMAN). The key is to set appropriate goals that build upon each other, and avoid the common human error of expecting a "perfect" outcome.

Those of us with physical limitations often dream of "perfect health" and being in a state where our body fully cooperates with everything we want it to do. We look at people who can run marathon after marathon without any significant health barriers and wonder why our bodies can't do that. However, we often overlook the majority of the population who do have some sort of physical limitation and allow it to limit the quality of their lives. We must explore what is possible given our body's limitations, and not be discouraged by an unrealistic expectation of "perfect health." Expectation is a huge driver of behavior. If your expectation is perfect health, but you can barely make it through your daily activities (for example, work, taking care of kids, etc.) without pain and discomfort, it's pretty hard to get motivated to work toward health improvement when the ultimate goal seems so far out of reach. However, if you set your initial expectation as feeling less exhausted at the end of the day, then your mind might be more willing to consider taking action toward that.

It is pretty hard to see beyond the limitations of our current health state. What we have to remember is that our current health state is simply a stepping stone to the next level. We need to keep searching for a way to get to the next level, to push those limits just a little further out. But WHY do you want to get to the next level of health and/or fitness? Only you can answer this question. If your expectation is that you can take steps toward feeling less exhausted at the end of the day, you need to ask yourself WHY that would matter. How will your life change if you're less exhausted all the time? What difference could you make in the lives of others if you had more energy?

The WHY must be powerful enough to drive you to seek the answers, take action, make sacrifices, suffer through the discomfort ... these are all necessary steps on the journey to "healthy." "Healthy" is a daily battle, not a final destination. Being human, chances are we will not fight this battle unless the goal and the WHY are very powerful for us. The prize for fighting the battle is a sense of accomplishment and satisfaction that we could never achieve without overcoming a physical limitation.

So think about your healthiest state as a journey, a battle that must be fought and embraced every day. It has nothing to do with "perfect health." It has everything to do with WHY you want to get to the next level of health and wellness.

Three

Step 3: Set Appropriate Goals

*Learn from the past, set vivid, detailed goals for
the future, and live in the only moment of time
over which you have any control: now.*
Denis Waitley

Before we get into goal setting (Step 3), I can't emphasize enough
the importance of first completing Step 2: Establish Your WHY.
Of course, goal setting is very important for making progress
in any aspect of your life. But have you ever wondered why you
seem so much more determined to follow through on some
goals than on others? That's likely because the goals you choose
to pursue with more fervor are more clearly aligned with your
life purpose and values. If you haven't yet articulated your
WHY—your life purpose—you'll have difficulty identifying
goals that are aligned with it! In that case, what transpires is
a process of trial and error, where you attempt to set goals
you think might be achievable, and your chances of following
through on each goal are random at best.

For example, my friend suggested that it would be fun to
learn how to scuba dive together. She is one of my closest
friends, with whom I love spending time. So I'm tempted to
say "yes" to her suggestion. However, as much as I value close
friends and physical activity, I have to say that scuba diving
is not on my bucket list. The main reason for this lies in the
fact that this type of activity requires significant effort to obtain a certification. Because my life purpose is "maximizing
potential," I like to engage in athletic undertakings that I can

practice frequently in order to improve my competence and feel like I'm making progress. Scuba diving doesn't meet those criteria for me, and neither would other activities that require upfront commitment and significant time investments without the opportunities for frequent practice. This doesn't apply to fun activities with my friends that I wouldn't view as requiring skill building, like going out for a hike and having a quality conversation in the process. That would be something I value deeply.

In other words, carefully select your goals based on how well they align with your life purpose. This increases the chances that you'll follow through with achieving the goals, which in turn rewards you with success. Since success breeds success, this process sets you up for an upward spiral of achievement.

> *Whether you believe you can do a thing or not,*
> *you are right.*
> **Henry Ford**

Sometimes it's hard to grasp the fact that goals are things that you CAN'T actually do today! So if you look at a challenge like running a marathon when all you can do is run 2 km before keeling over, of course your reaction is "I can't do that." Because you CAN'T ... at least, not today. And that's the key. So you can believe you can't, and simply close the door on the goal, or you can believe you can't *today*, and begin taking steps in the direction that will increase the chances of getting there in the future. There's a huge difference in mindset between "I can't do that" and "I can't do that *today*."

I remember completing my second sprint triathlon (750 m open-water swim, 25 km bike, and 7 km run), when my husband suggested we should set a goal of doing an Olympic distance triathlon the next year. This would involve a 1,500 m open-water swim, 40 km bike, and 10 km run. My first reaction was

"I don't know ... I don't think I can do 1,500 m in open water. I just struggled to do 750 m." The problem here is that I was basing my opinion on the skills and abilities I possessed at that moment. The key is to set the goal, then figure out a way to be able to do it.

The next time you're considering a seemingly impossible goal, try responding with something like this: "I'm not sure if I can do that, but I'm willing to try. What steps would I need to take in order to be able to achieve that?" Whether we can actually accomplish something is often more of a choice than we think. It's a choice of staying in our current state or comfort zone versus putting in the effort required to move up to a new level.

As for the Olympic triathlon challenge, my husband's reaction was, "We just need to become better swimmers!" So we began taking steps toward becoming stronger swimmers, joining an instructional swimming program and increasing our swim distances that winter. Not only did I eventually conquer the Olympic distance race, but it gave me the courage to set my sights on the next distance, a half-iron triathlon, which then led me to my first IRONMAN event in 2013. Once a goal is achieved, it serves as a stepping stone to the next, bigger goal.

Remember, success breeds success. Break the big goals down into achievable steps and celebrate accomplishments along the way, no matter how small.

Guidelines for Choosing Appropriate Goals

A good rule of thumb for effective goal setting is to articulate SMART goals.

S = Specific—Can you clearly articulate the goal?

M = Measurable—In order to be measurable, the goal can't be vague like "I want to feel better" or "I want to lose weight." Specific and measurable would be something like "I want to climb ten steps without having to stop for a break."

A = Achievable—You can see your way to achieving the goal. Maybe not today or tomorrow, but your mind can wrap itself around attaining it within a reasonable timeframe. You also need to keep in mind that the goal must be under your control. In other words, you can't set a goal to eliminate toxins in the global environment, but you can control the choices you make in contributing to or countering your local environment's toxicity.

R = Relevant—The goal must mean something to you. In other words, it must be aligned with your values and your WHY. Without that alignment, your odds of success are greatly diminished. You must be able to answer "Why am I working toward this goal?" with something that is personally very meaningful and powerful.

T = Time-sensitive—You need to create some sort of urgency in order to drive momentum toward achieving the goal.

This past year, having not had the spectre of an IRONMAN hanging over me, it's been rather challenging to keep myself motivated to work out. I said to my husband, "I don't know why it seems like such a chore to work out these days. I'm having trouble getting motivated."

To which he responded, "That's because you're not scared!"

Once I processed what he meant, I realized he was absolutely right. I don't have a looming deadline for which I need to have a specific level of training completed. Immediately after signing up for the IRONMAN event, I had a brief moment of panic but shifted quickly to consulting the training guide and booking workouts in my calendar. There was a fire under my butt for those eight months from the date of sign up to the date of the race. Having a deadline is incredibly powerful. It means commitment. Just take a deep breath, push through the fear, and set a specific date by which you must accomplish your goal. Make it a firm date, ideally backed by financial commitment, like paying an entry or registration fee.

The one criterion I believe lacks emphasis in the SMART acronym is that of finding ways to ensure your commitment. A few ideas for this would include sharing your goal with as many people as possible, or committing significant resources toward achieving the goal. By sharing your intent with others, you commit yourself socially—no one wants to lose face by not following through on public commitments. Additionally, the act of committing resources (such as money) will lead to greater commitment on your part. One example is to sign up for an event that involves a participation fee, and then figure out how you're going to be ready for the event. As noted above, this can also be linked to the time sensitivity of the goal.

According to studies done on healthy aging, "cultivating a sense of progress" is one of the key habits found among older individuals with above-average longevity who have managed to maintain above-average vitality and happiness into their later years (Bruce Grierson, *What Makes Olga Run*). This is directly linked to setting appropriate goals. If you're comparing your current capabilities to what you were able to do when younger and healthier, you're setting yourself up for disappointment and inaction. Interestingly, those of us who struggled for years in our youth might be at an advantage in terms of healthy aging. Now that I'm healthier and stronger than ever, I can set goals that I was never able to set in my twenties and thirties!

It's never too late to set progressive goals. It's just a matter of setting yourself up for progress by adjusting the yardstick.

Adjusting the Yardstick for Maximum Motivation

I stopped playing tennis in 2008 after playing on and off for twenty-nine years. I found it too hard on my body, and after twelve years of limited practice due to chronic injuries, my level of play had become very unsatisfying when compared to the levels I had achieved in my prime. I was accepting that I could no longer do activities with the intensity that I wanted. Since I wanted to stay as active and fit as I could be, swimming presented a lower-risk option.

So I decided to follow my friend to a swimming class one evening after work. Although I "knew" how to swim from having taken lessons as a child, I couldn't finish a lap of front crawl without gasping for air! After struggling through and barely completing half of the laps that the rest of the class completed, I felt exhausted, yet strangely motivated to try again. With a few tips from the instructor over the next several classes, I began to understand how I could swim more efficiently and therefore be less tired after each lap. These glimmers of hope that my stroke could improve kept me going back.

My friend and I then began discussing the possibility of doing a short triathlon someday. I was intrigued. When I found the sports medicine clinic that changed my life in 2009 and started to feel like I wasn't necessarily trapped in a stiff, sore, and chronically injured body, I signed up for my first "Sprint" triathlon. My goals were as follows:

- Don't get injured.
- Finish.
- Don't be last in my age group.

These were all pretty achievable and measurable goals. I struggled through that first race, but met all three goals. It was the most empowering feeling I had ever had. When I signed up to do the same race the following year, I improved my time and my placement within my age group. Since 2010, I've conquered longer and longer triathlon distances and improved my placement within my age group. This is so incredibly motivating! That's when I realized, it's great to start at the bottom, because there's nowhere to go but up! I am driven to work on my swim, bike, and run techniques as well as my endurance because I want to improve, and there is lots of room for improvement. I have no expectations of being good or better than others at triathlon; I simply want to keep improving on my own performances.

I contrast this with tennis. Having been a very competent varsity and club-level player in my teens and twenties, it was difficult to stay motivated when my performance level kept declining with the limitations imposed by my chronic pain condition. I strongly encourage you, as you move forward in your Health Champion journey, to select new (appropriate) activities that intrigue you, and get ready to be motivated at the prospect of continuous improvement.

> *What you get by achieving your goals is not as important as what you become by achieving your goals.*
> **Henry David Thoreau**

As much as I like the previous quote by Thoreau, I would modify it slightly to the following: "What you get by achieving your goals is not as important as what you become by *working toward* achieving your goals."

While your goal is a specific and measurable outcome (an

example was my goal to complete an IRONMAN triathlon), there is a process that needs to occur in order to reach it. That process will inevitably be fraught with both predictable and unpredictable obstacles. Sometimes it will feel like the goal is eluding you. What's important is that you stop periodically to appreciate how far you've come, merely because you set the goal in the first place.

There were several points in time when I doubted my ability to show up for the IRONMAN event. There were injuries and other obstacles reducing my ability to train. However, the process of moving toward that goal made me the healthiest and fittest I had ever dreamt I could become. The most important result of setting the goal to complete an IRONMAN was the progress I made in finding additional solutions to address my chronic pain condition, so that I could have a chance at completing the race. Just appreciating this fact was a huge victory. I knew deep down that if I couldn't complete the race in 2013, I would eventually find a way to complete one in another year, because of all the health progress I was making.

During the "dark years," when I was still searching for ways to manage the pain, my goal was to be able to carry my children upstairs. At the time, they only weighed 25 to 35 pounds. As I thought about what I needed to do in order for this to happen, I realized I needed to get stronger, despite the pain issue. This eventually led me to an exceptional strength coach, who not only worked with me on building up my strength, but who was knowledgeable enough to do this in a gradual way so as to avoid aggravating the chronic injuries that had been plaguing me for years. Not only that; she began delving into potential causes for my underlying condition, and bringing in other health experts to address the root of the problem.

So my small goal of wanting to be strong enough to carry my kids eventually led me to become strong enough (over four years) to complete an IRONMAN triathlon! I think a key factor here is to continue setting goals, no matter what. Not only do goals keep you moving forward, but the mere process of moving forward can lead you to stumble upon hidden clues and treasures that can pave the way for exponential improvement.

Take a few moments to answer the following questions:

1. What goal could you set that would be a catalyst to help you move toward your optimal condition? Hint: a goal is something you can't accomplish today, and you're not even sure you can ever accomplish it ... but it is aligned with your purpose and the attempt to achieve it is worthy. Something in the back of your mind says, "Maybe there's a chance" when you think of this goal. Note that I'm encouraging you to push yourself to "think big"; however, the goal must be achievable (remember the "A" in SMART). This means your mind must be able to imagine there is at least a possibility of achieving it.

2. In looking at the goal you listed in #1 just above, ask yourself, "What is the first thing I need to do in order to get there?" Are there certain sub-goals or milestones that could be reached along the way? Break down your "big" goal into smaller sub-goals or milestones.

3. How could you celebrate success as you achieve each of the smaller sub-goals?

Don't delay in setting new goals for yourself as your health improves.

Set the Goal, Then Let Go

One of the key things I learned during my years in sales was the importance of disassociating myself from the outcome of a negotiation. It's a bit counterintuitive, but the less you're married to a specific outcome, the better the chance that your negotiation will have a successful outcome for you and the other party(ies) involved.

In applying this concept to setting goals, think about your emotional self negotiating with your rational self in the process of goal setting. When the goal seems daunting and almost un-achievable, your emotional self (which has the desire) needs to be able to trick your rational self into believing that you really don't care whether you get there or not. Set the big overarching goal, tell your rational self it would be nice but not critical to get there, then start breaking it down into much smaller short-term goals that your rational brain can accept as "doable." As you smash through each small goal, your confidence will build and eventually your rational brain will begin to accept the pos-sibility that the "impossible" goal set forth by your emotional brain might not be that impossible after all.

How I wrapped my mind around signing up for an IRONMAN event might help you to embrace this concept of setting the big goal and letting it go before your rational brain stops you. After completing a half-iron triathlon in 2012, I began to dream a little about what it would take to do an IRONMAN race. Every time my mind wandered in that direction, the rational part of my brain would weigh in with "No way. You can't do that." But the vision of completing an IRONMAN race as a way to shout my Health Champion message out to the world became emotionally compelling. My emotional brain wanted to go for it, but the rational side kept fighting back with reasons why it was absolutely not possible for me to go the full distance, given my health history.

So I simply said to myself, "Why not sign up and follow a training program? Let's see where it leads. If I don't succeed, the worst that can happen is that I get even fitter and stronger. And if I get injured in the process, I now know how to deal with any training injury that might pop up."

In essence, I was tricking my rational brain by telling it that it didn't matter whether I could complete the IRONMAN or not. I was just going to start down the training path and see where it led.

First step, sign up for the race before it sells out. Second step, pull out the training manual and fill your calendar with workouts for the next couple of months. Third step, call your strength coach and ask her to tweak your strength training program so as to complement the IRONMAN training plan. And so it went, one step at a time, dealing with every hurdle as it came, reminding myself that simply being in a position to train for this incredible event was a victory. Showing up and completing the race would be bonuses. This was my ploy to get around that pesky, doubtful, disbelieving rational brain.

SECTION I—SUMMARY

In Section I, Steps 1 through 3 laid the groundwork for this pivotal phase of the Health Champion program. Please go through and ensure that you can confidently check the boxes below and confirm you've established your Health Champion mindset. Before moving to the action phase of Part II, it's important to have a clear destination and roadmap of where you are headed.

Step 1: Identify What's Holding You Back

☐ I've become aware of at least one deeply held belief, expectation, or behavior that could be playing a role in keeping me "stuck" in my current situation.

☐ I believe that there's more I can do to help myself advance on my Health Champion journey, in order to achieve more in life.

Step 2: Determine Your WHY

☐ I've devoted sufficient time to arriving at my WHY, and it is a purpose that involves positively impacting the lives of others.

☐ I've "peeled back the onion" in identifying my WHY, by drilling down and asking myself "Why would it matter?" several times.

☐ My WHY statement is specific, personal, and evokes much emotion when I articulate it.

Step 3: Set Appropriate Goals

☐ I've identified one key goal for improving my health, which is aligned with my WHY.

☐ I've broken down the larger goal into smaller ones and applied the SMART acronym to each:

- ☐ Specific
- ☐ Measurable
- ☐ Achievable
- ☐ Relevant
- ☐ Time-sensitive
- ☐ I know exactly what actions I can take today and tomorrow to begin moving toward my goal.
- ☐ I know how I will celebrate each milestone along the way.

SECTION II

Build and Leverage Your Health Champion Team

At this point, you will have done the following:

- Identified some of the issues holding you back and keeping you from achieving your full potential.
- Envisioned your greater purpose, your WHY. This is the "force" that will pull you forward, and allow you to muster the strength to face the adversity that you will inevitably face as you move forward in your journey.
- Set goals that are aligned with your purpose, which will be challenging to achieve, but that are worthy of the effort required to reach them.

Now that you've established a deliberate, purpose-driven and goal-oriented mindset about your health, you're ready to start building and leveraging your Health Champion team. This means surrounding yourself with the right people and making the most of the knowledge, experience, and expertise held by these people. You need an inner circle of supporters, a broader social network that can be a source of valuable information, health professionals with a problem-solving mindset—regardless of the letters beside their names—and a budget dedicated to your new health venture.

Defining Effective Problem-Solving

You will notice that I mention problem-solving a lot in this section. So this is probably a good place to discuss what is meant by effective problem-solving. One of the best known and most remarkable problem solvers in history was Albert Einstein. He is often quoted as having said that if he had one hour to save the world he would spend fifty-five minutes defining the problem and only five minutes finding the solution. In other words, the most important step in problem-solving is to clearly define the problem in the first place. What usually happens is that as soon as we have a problem to work on, we're so eager to get to solutions that we neglect spending any time refining it. This applies both to us and to our health professionals.

Once the problem is clearly defined and understood, not only will your solutions be more abundant and of higher quality, but you'll achieve them much, much more easily. Most importantly, you'll be motivated by the fact that you're tackling a worthwhile problem. In my personal example, I've figured out that a key part of my chronic pain problem is the lack of absorption of key nutrients by my small intestine. This is because of damage inflicted by foods to which my body is intolerant—namely glutenous grains. Now that the problem is clearly defined, the solutions are straightforward. I avoid the foods that are causing the problem and load up on foods that enable better myofascial function (see Chapter 10 for details). Had I been able to spend more time upfront digging into the causes of my pain (rather than throwing haphazard band-aid solutions at them), I could have solved my pain and recovered in a much shorter time.

I believe so strongly in the need for better problem-solving in healthcare. Not only is this necessary at the health professional level, but as the Chief Problem Solver for your health challenges, it is important that you sharpen your own problem-solving skills. Your efforts, combined with those of good problem-solving health professionals, are much more likely to contribute to uncovering effective solutions for your particular situation.

The good news is that using different perspectives to clearly define a problem is a skill that can be learned and developed. A good place to find strategies for problem definition is the world of mathematics and science. Below are some strategies for problem definition taken from my science background and some internet research on the subject.[12] I've added some healthcare examples to help you look at things differently. Can you apply any of these to your particular health problem?

Strategy #1: Rephrase the Problem

If someone at work asked you to brainstorm "ways to increase your productivity," how many ideas would come to mind? What if the exercise were rephrased as "ways to make your job easier." I'm going to guess you could come up with many more suggestions when phrased the latter way.

The choice of words can play a major role in how we perceive a problem. In the example above, "be productive" might seem like a sacrifice you're doing for the company, while "make your job easier" may be more like something you're doing for your own benefit, but from which the company also benefits. In the end, the problem is still the same, but the feelings—and the points of view associated with each of them—are different.

Play freely with the problem statement, rewording it several times. For a methodical approach, take single words and substitute variations. For example, when considering the phrase "increase activity," try replacing "increase" with "attract, develop, extend, repeat" and see how your perception of the problem

---

[12] litemind.com; and
www.une.edu.au/about-une/academic-schools/bcss/news-and-events/psychology-community-activities/over-fifty-problem-solving-strategies-explained; and
teacher.scholastic.com/lessonrepro/lessonplans/steppro.htm

changes. A rich vocabulary plays an important role here, so you probably want to use a thesaurus for this exercise.

Strategy #2: Expose and Challenge Assumptions

Every problem—no matter how simple it may appear—comes with a long list of assumptions attached. Many of these assumptions may be inaccurate and could make your problem statement inadequate or even misguided.

The first step to get rid of bad assumptions is to make them explicit. Write a list and expose as many assumptions as you can—especially those that may seem the most obvious and "untouchable." In my case, the assumption was that doctors and prescriptions would hold the answer to my condition.

That in itself brings more clarity to the problem at hand. But go further and test each assumption for validity. Think in ways that present the assumptions and their consequences as invalid. What you will find may surprise you. Many of those bad assumptions are self-imposed, and with just a bit of scrutiny you are able to safely drop them.

For example, suppose you're about to enter the taxi business. One of your assumptions might be, "Taxi drivers have to know their way around the city." While such an assumption may seem true at first, try challenging it and maybe you'll find some very interesting business models, such as New York City designating certain taxis for locals only—the drivers are new to the city and don't know their way around well, but local inhabitants can direct them.

As a healthcare example, what if you threw away the assumption that doctors know how to diagnose health problems? What would this lead you to do? Perhaps you might need to be better prepared for your appointments? Maybe you need to ask questions to try and lead the physician into problem-solving?

Or throw out any and all assumptions you've made to date

about your current health problem. Don't hold back. If you've broken your leg, question the assumption that you won't be walking for several weeks. How does that change the way you look at your rehabilitation program?

Strategy #3: Make It Bigger

Each problem is a small piece of a greater problem. This is called exploring the problem at different "altitudes."

If you feel you're overwhelmed with details or looking at a problem too narrowly, look at it from a more general perspective. In order to make your problem more general, ask questions like, "What's this a part of?" or "What's this an example of?" or "What's the intention behind this?"

Another approach that helps a lot in getting a more general view of a problem is replacing words in the problem statement with hypernyms. "Hypernyms" are words that have a broader meaning than the given word. For example, a hypernym of "health" is "welfare." A great, free tool for finding hypernyms for a given word is Princeton University's WordNet.[13] Just search for a word and click on the "S" label before the word definitions.

Strategy #4: Make It Smaller

If each problem is part of a greater problem, it also means that each problem is composed of many smaller problems. It turns out that decomposing a problem into many smaller problems— each of them more specific than the original—can also provide greater insights about it.

Making the problem smaller or more specific is especially useful if you find the problem overwhelming or daunting. Some of the typical questions you can ask to make a problem

---

[13]wordnetweb.princeton.edu/perl/webwn

more specific are, "What are the parts of this?" or "What are examples of this?"

Just as in "Strategy #3: Make It Bigger," word substitution can also come to great use here. The class of words that are useful here are hyponyms, words that are stricter in meaning than the given one. For example, two hyponyms of "worry" are "imposition" and "burden." WordNet can also help you with finding hyponyms.

Strategy #5: Find Multiple Perspectives

Before rushing to solve a problem, always make sure you look at it from different perspectives. Looking at it with different eyes is a great way to have instant insight on new, overlooked directions.

For example, if you're trying to reduce pain, view this problem from the point of view of, say, a family member. For example, from the family member's viewpoint, this may be a matter of you being able to participate in specific activities with them. Maybe presenting the problem from this perspective can trigger you and/or your health professionals to look at different solutions focused on helping you regain functionality, which extends beyond simply controlling the pain (the band-aid solution). Perhaps this even leads you down new avenues, toward solving the underlying issue behind the pain.

Rewrite your problem statement many times, each time using one of these different perspectives. How would your friends see this problem? Your employer? Your employees? Your grandparents? Also, imagine how people in various roles would frame the problem. How would a teacher see it? An Olympic athlete? Try to find the differences and similarities on how the different roles would deal with your problem.

Strategy #6: Use Various Language Constructs

There isn't a magic formula for properly crafting a problem statement, but there are some language constructs that can help make it more effective.

Assume there are many potential solutions. An excellent way to start a problem statement is "In what ways might I ...?" This expression is much superior to "How can I ...?" The former indicates that there's a multitude of solutions, and not just one or none. As simple as this sounds, the feeling of expectancy helps your brain find solutions.

Make it positive. Negative sentences require a lot more brain power to process and may slow you down—or even derail your train of thought. Positive statements also help you find the real goal behind the problem and, as such, are much more motivating. For example, instead of finding ways to "quit smoking," you may find that "increase my energy and live longer" are much more worthwhile goals.

Frame your problem in the form of a question. Our brain loves questions. If the question is powerful and engaging, our brains will do everything within their reach to answer it. We just can't help it. Our brains will start working on the problem immediately and keep working in the background, even when we're not aware of it.

Strategy #7: Make It Engaging

In addition to using effective language constructs, it's important to come up with a problem statement that truly excites you so you're in the best frame of mind for creatively tackling the problem. If the problem looks too dull for you, invest the time adding vigor to it while still keeping it genuine. Make it enticing. Your brain will thank (and reward) you later.

It's one thing to "feel better" (boring); it is another to "have the energy to play with my kids." One thing is to "create a personal development blog"; another completely different statement is to "empower readers to live fully." Note how this ties into your WHY. Your mind will be driven to defining the problem and solving it if the problem is framed around something that excites you—your life purpose.

Strategy #8: Look at the Problem Backwards

One trick that usually helps when you're stuck with a problem is turning it on its head. If you want to win, find out what would make you lose. If you are struggling finding ways to "feel better," find ways to feel worse instead. Then, all you need to do is reverse your answers. For example, if my challenge is to figure out how to get better at running, when running causes foot pain, I will come up with how my running could get worse. My running would get worse if I never ran at all. It would also get worse if I ran so much that I destroyed my feet. When I turn it around, it makes me think, "How can I run without running?" This leads me to think of activities that I can substitute for running without causing me foot pain. Water running (running in a pool while suspended with a water belt) and the elliptical trainer are two great substitutes that train most of the running muscles without necessarily causing the foot pain that comes from the impact of running. This seemingly convoluted method may not seem intuitive at first, but turning a problem on its head can uncover rather obvious solutions to the original problem.

Strategy #9: Gather Facts

Investigate causes and circumstances of the problem. Probe details about it—such as its origins and basis. Especially when you have a problem that's too vague, investigating facts is usually more productive than trying to solve the problem right away.

For example, if you have a headache, you might want to consider additional details like the following: Where exactly does it hurt in my head? Is it a constant, dull ache, or is it sharp and intermittent? Where was I and what was I doing when the symptoms started? In a discussion with a health professional, the more details you provide the better he or she will be able to help sort out the cause of the problem so that the best solution can be uncovered.

Be curious when gathering facts. Not only do you need to ask yourself questions; you also need to ask other stakeholders like family members and friends. And by asking questions of your health professionals, you can work as a team to define your particular problem more descriptively. It is said that a well-defined problem is halfway to being solved; one could argue that a perfectly defined problem is not a problem anymore.

When you start paying more attention to how you define your problems, you'll probably find that it is much harder than solving them. But you'll also find that the payoff is well worth the effort. But isn't that usually the case? When we invest ourselves in tackling the hard stuff, the rewards are that much more satisfying.

Let's get to work building and leveraging the Health Champion team that, with your committed problem-solving efforts, can help you get closer to living your life to its fullest potential.

Four

Step 4: Develop and Use Your Social Support Network

When we give cheerfully and accept gratefully, everyone is blessed.
Maya Angelou

This step has three components: identifying supporters, leveraging the knowledge and experience of your entire social network, and taking action.

First, you need to identify supporters within your inner circle and maximize the time you spend with them, as opposed to those who are judgmental, negative, or unsupportive. Supporters are people who might not have any suggestions or answers for you, but they will be there for you no matter what approach you choose for tackling your health issues. Second, make the most of your entire social network by allowing them the opportunity to share their knowledge and experiences with you. Most people genuinely want to help. If they have any information whatsoever that might lead to improving your life, they will share it. The only requirement is that you communicate your health challenges to them and give them permission to help you. Third, it is your responsibility to follow through and act on the information you receive when someone shares a potential lead that has even a remote chance of contributing to your health improvement.

Identifying Your Supporters

One of the many moments in my twenty-three years of marriage when I knew I picked the right guy came when we were going through infertility treatments. After several failed IVF (In Vitro Fertilization) attempts, I was pretty demoralized. Rod's response was simply, "We just keep trying until we're successful." Sure enough, a few years later we were successful at least in part because his positive attitude encouraged me to keep searching for an answer. We now have two beautiful daughters.

In 2011 when I planned to do my first Olympic distance triathlon (which starts with a 1,500 m swim), I barely finished the 500 m swim in the first warm-up race that season. With only six weeks to go, I was so discouraged. I asked Rod, "How can I possibly do 1,500 m at the Olympic race?"

Rod's response was simply, "We will find a place to do some open-water training." He identified a nearby quarry where many triathletes trained, never faltering in his belief that I would be able to do the longer distances if I just practiced more. The issue was more one of intimidation by open water, because I could swim up to 2,000 m in a pool at that point.

Thanks to Rod's positive attitude and the affiliation with my new inspiring friends at the quarry, I conquered the Olympic triathlon in 2011, and progressed through to a 3,800 m open-water swim at my IRONMAN race in 2013.

The key to identifying supportive friends lies in the fact that they never question your efforts to set and meet your goals. They might not relate to your goals, or understand why you want to achieve these goals, but they are there for you, wishing you the best and cheering for your success. When I told my friend MT that I was planning to run a marathon in 2013 as part of my training plan for the IRONMAN, her first response was, "I'm there." She literally meant she would be there ... not only cheering for me but running it with me, seeing me through those brutal final 12 km (out of 42 km). The night before the marathon, she gave me a card that featured a quote attributed to Winston Churchill: "Never, never, never give up." Whether she ran the race with me or not, she was there for me.

Take a moment to list the five people with whom you spend the most time on a regular basis. Beside each of their names, make a note about how they would respond if you shared with them an outlandish goal, for example, "Within two years, I want to be able to climb Mount Everest." Would you be hearing things like, "Amazing. How can I help you get there?" or is it more like, "Yeah right, don't be ridiculous."

1. ____
2. ____
3. ____
4. ____
5. ____

Select the one or two members of your inner circle who are most supportive and think of ways that you can increase your time spent with them, while gradually reducing your exposure to those who are unsupportive.

If you can't identify one person within your inner circle that you can count on as a supporter, how could you begin to form at least one supportive relationship in your life? Can you look into joining organizations related to your passions or activities that you really enjoy? What about a support group whose focus is truly to provide positive support to members reaching for new heights? Do you currently have friends or acquaintances that you've identified as positive and supportive, to whom you could reach out and increase the time you spend with them, essentially "transplanting" them into your inner circle and crowding out the non-supportive relationships?

It might be difficult at times, but you need to distance yourself from anyone who can't be supportive of your efforts to reach higher goals that are meaningful to you. In many cases, this means distancing yourself from people you did not choose to be in your life, even if that includes certain family members. As a respected colleague once said to me, "You are only required to honor your family members, not to love them or go out of your way to spend time with them." So fulfill your family obligations, but choose wisely when it comes to investing your time with people.

If you really believe that reducing the amount of time spent in the presence of negative or judgmental people is not an option for you (at least not to the degree that it would make a difference for you), you can begin working on your resilience in terms of limiting the negative impact these people are having on you. In chapter six of her book *Feel the Fear and Do It Anyway*, Susan Jeffers, Ph.D. talks about handling situations in which family members and friends don't appear to appreciate your personal growth journey. She illustrates how to turn negative interactions into win-win interactions. An example would be when a family member tells you that you can't succeed. Rather than responding defensively or lashing out at them (lose-lose), you could respond with something like, "I appreciate your concern. I realize there are risks involved in what I want to do, but I have enough faith in myself that I know I can handle the challenges that come up. I'd really like it if you could have more faith in me also."

Jeffers also recommends the book *Aikido in Everyday Life* by Terry Dobson and Victor Miller (Blue Snake Books, 1994) on the subject of nonaggressive self-defense. Self-defense is essentially what we're dealing with when those around us seem determined to knock down our attempts to move forward and improve our lives. I call it self-preservation. Either way, it's critical to reduce our exposure to their negative assaults and to arm ourselves with strategies to lessen the impact of the blows.

A less obvious but just as damaging situation occurs when you're surrounded with people who appear to be supportive, but are continuously imposing their own ideal goals or targets on you. You might think you're doing well avoiding the overtly negative influences in your life, but are you substituting them with others who keep pushing you toward their own vision of what's "right" for you? It's critical to find at least one close connection who is non-judgmental and simply supports you in your quest to reach higher goals that matter to you.

Although this isn't a book about coaching, consider the fact that a good coach is someone who takes the position that you have all the qualities you need to reach your full potential. The coach's role is to help you identify your strengths, hold you accountable for taking action on what you already know you need to do, and support you through the process in ways that are directed by your preferences. If you feel like you're not getting this type of unconditional support and empowerment from your existing relationships, I encourage you to find a good coach to help you through the process of uncovering your potential.

Associate Not Only With Positive and Supportive People, but With Inspiring People

In addition to that small inner circle of supporters, look for organizations, groups, or individuals who are achieving goals similar to the ones you want to achieve, but at a much higher level. When Rod and I joined the quarry in Caledon, Ontario to practice our open-water swimming, little did we know the group was led by Barrie Shepley, former Olympic triathlon coach. Some of the athletes training there are incredibly high-performing triathletes, including Olympic contenders and national champions. Had we known this upfront, we might not have signed up to swim there because of the intimidation factor. Now in our fifth year of training at the quarry and associating with high-level triathletes (as well as lots of others like us, just looking to do their personal best and finish the race), we realize it was the best thing we ever did. Even more important than having the quarry available for open-water practice is the motivation and inspiration that comes with being a part of this group of athletes. There is definitely a positive impact on goal setting and performance when we're in the midst of high-performing athletes versus being on our own.

In 2013, after my first early morning swim of the season (6:30 a.m.) at the quarry, I went back to my car, walking through the mud (the ground was very wet and mucky). As I tried to turn my car around to leave the quarry area, my tires got stuck in the mud! I was about ten inches deep with my front tires, which were just spinning, throwing mud everywhere. The only two people left at the quarry were national elite triathletes Sean Bechtel and Taylor Reid. They didn't give a second thought to helping me try to get out, going as far as digging mud with their bare hands! They just about had me out, when I ran out of gas! I said to them "I should have just gone to the pool." To which Taylor replied "No, because then you wouldn't have a story to tell."

Since that moment, I've looked at difficult and "bad luck" situations in a whole new light. I will often stop myself when my thoughts and emotions start to slide into the negative and tell myself, "This is giving me another story to tell." I am so grateful for having the opportunity to spend time with such positive influences.

How can you set yourself up to be in the presence of positive, supportive, and inspiring influences? I ask you this question because there are some fascinating social science research findings indicating that other people have an influence on our self-regulation. Although it is a subconscious process, the impact of others on our own emotional state and level of performance has been measured. As much as you wanted to deny your parents' opinions about certain friends being "bad influences," there might have been more merit to these opinions than you would like to acknowledge.

At a recent conference, renowned psychologist, public speaker, and author Todd Kashdan shared some incredible research related to the impact of social relationships on our ability to perform at our highest levels. The findings indicate that when we feel surrounded and supported by people we trust, our ability to set goals, take action, and stay focused improves significantly. This applies even when we're exposed to photos of people we trust. The closer and more trusted the individual, the better the brain can "let go" and focus on the task ahead.

Think about these specific findings of the research: we will adjust our goals, depending on the facial expressions of people we know and trust. Our commitment and performance toward achieving a goal is directly related to the attitude of our trusted social network toward that goal. In fact, even the thought of someone we love and trust will significantly impact our goal setting and performance.[14] So surround yourself (physically and virtually) with those you trust and love, and your chances of reaching new levels of health and fulfillment are increased. Whose image is on *your* screensaver?

Leveraging Your Social Network

Social science research points to the fact that we can acquire additional cognitive resources by simply associating with others we trust.[15] These individuals are not necessarily members of our "inner circle." They can be any combination

---

[14]Shah, James. "The motivational looking glass: How significant others implicitly affect goal appraisals." *Journal of Personality and Social Psychology*, Vol 85(3), Sep 2003, 424-439.
[15]Beckes L and Coan J. "Social baseline theory: The role of proximity in emotion and economy of action." *Social & Personality Psychology Compass*, 2011, 976-988.

of friends, colleagues, respected acquaintances, or family members with whom you maintain a stable social relationship. They are referred to in psychology and other social sciences as being part of your "tribe." According to research by British anthropologist Robin Dunbar, an ideal tribe size for our brains to outsource resources to and to function more productively is about 150.[16] Think about your expanded social network. Who is in it? Are there people you trust and feel confident about, knowing that they "have your back"? Are there people who offer you inspiration?

The ostrich presents a great example of social outsourcing. When feeding in groups, ostriches will enjoy a much more efficient and fulfilling feeding experience than when feeding alone. When alone, the ostrich has to continually pop its head up to look for the presence of predators. It expends much brainpower and energy on stress related to self-preservation rather than on searching for and eating food to thrive. When in a group, the ostriches will trust that at any one time, one bird will have its head up and, therefore, they can relax and allocate more brainpower to feeding. Are you continuously expending energy on self-preservation, or are you working on thriving?

The idea is for you to "spread the load" in terms of dealing with your health challenges and leverage your social network to efficiently arrive at solutions. You want to be able to let go of unproductive brain processes (for example, those processes being allocated to stress and worry about your current condition) in order to allocate those brain resources to problem-solving. In addition, most people want to help when presented with someone else's challenge. Unless you share information with your network and make it clear you're open to their suggestions, you'll never discover what they know or what experiences they've had that you could benefit from. Be selective,

---

[16]R.I.M. Dunbar, (1993), Coevolution of neocortical size, group size and language in humans, *Behavioral and Brain Sciences* 16 (4): 681–735.

but don't be afraid to share your challenges with your tribe. You'd be surprised where this can lead. Are you giving your network the opportunities and the permissions to offer you helpful information?

Now that you've considered who you're going to spend more or less time with, and with whom you're going to share your health challenges, there is one last critical component to this step. It is your responsibility to follow all leads offered to you. You don't know what you don't know, so if someone offers you information that doesn't make sense to you, check it out anyway. You can always rule it out later.

When I think back to my infertility experience, all three components of "Develop and Use Your Social Support Network" were in play, and all three were critical to our success in conceiving our daughters. Firstly, I had my close supporter in Rod. His mantra was, "Whatever it takes." Secondly, I shared my struggles with selected friends and colleagues, and during one of these conversations, I was directed to a Centers for Disease Control and Prevention website that held some remarkable facts about the vast difference in success rates between fertility clinics across the country. Thirdly, I acted upon my colleague's recommendation to review the data and I contacted Dr. Schoolcraft, a fertility specialist whose success rate was more than double that of the doctor I was seeing at the time.

You can't underestimate the power of your social network as part of your Health Champion team. Build it, leverage it, and take action.

Five

Step 5: Select and Challenge the Right Health Professionals

Think outside the square. Think for yourself. Don't just follow the herd. Think multidisciplinary! Problems, by definition, cross many academic disciplines.
Lucas Remmerswaal, *The A-Z of 13 Habits:*
Inspired by Warren Buffett

At this point, you will have started the process of building your Health Champion team by identifying your social support network—those who are going to lift you up, cheer you on, and support you in your drive toward reaching your goals and achieving your optimal state of wellness. And you've committed to sharing your challenges with your "tribe" or broader network, in order to gain from their experiences and their insights.

Now you're ready to uncover the resources and build the Health Professional part of the team that will help you move forward in your journey. It is critical that you start out with the mindset that you are the one in charge of discovering the solutions to the health challenges that are keeping you from living your ideal life. You are now the Chief Problem Solver for your health challenges. This does not mean you need to go out and earn an M.D. diploma! What it does mean is that you need to know how to discover and get the most benefit from the health resources that exist out there.

You have the right to demand a problem-solving partnership

from the members of your health team. You must be prepared to advocate for yourself, and let them know when you're not satisfied with the answers you're getting. If you don't feel qualified or capable of self-advocacy, find a member of your social network who is willing to help you prepare for appointments or have these conversations on your behalf or simply be there with you for moral support. Another option is to hire a health coach who can help you build your self-advocacy capabilities and steer you in the right direction.

Your rights to being treated as a partner and being respected for self-advocating in healthcare come with responsibilities. You have the responsibility to be as prepared and informed as possible when you attend an appointment. This is your part of the equation. You will not get the most from your healthcare appointments if you're not informed or prepared. Being prepared means you will have done the following:

- You've compiled a list of symptoms and any related circumstances that could shed light on the cause of the symptoms.
- You've prepared questions in advance, and are ready to ask as many questions as it takes to be satisfied that the health professional is going down the right path in terms of diagnosis and treatment.
- You've done some research, either by speaking to others who have suffered similar symptoms, by searching on the internet, and/or by asking for input from anyone in your social network who has some sort of healthcare background, or who might know someone with a healthcare background.

If you think about it, what I'm suggesting in terms of preparing for healthcare appointments is comparable to the degree of preparation you would put into a large purchase like a car or an expensive appliance. For your largest purchases like vacations or real estate, think about the amount of research and preparation you put in. Perhaps you want to take a step back and consider the value of a healthy life compared to these types of purchases. I know we've been taught to defer to physicians when it comes to health knowledge, and it's likely they will always have more specific health knowledge than we do. However, there is no way to leverage the full power of their knowledge to our maximum benefit unless we do our homework and work with the medical professional to solve our unique problem.

I believe our biggest mistake in dealing with health issues is having the expectation that the "experts" hold the answers, and that we just need to bring our problem to them to get a resolution.

There are a number of issues to take into consideration when dealing with health professionals:

- The letters beside their names will not tell you if they are good at what they do or if they will be effective at solving your problem.
- A top expert in his/her field might have the best grasp of the medical literature, but they don't have insight into the nuances of what's been happening in your body. They need your input in order to tailor their knowledge to address your particular situation most effectively.
- Depending on your particular health issues, the professional(s) who can help you the most might not be found in the mainstream medical system.
- Health professionals who are open to working collaboratively with other health professionals and who embrace a holistic, multidisciplinary approach are generally valuable and are more likely to be problem solvers determined to help you get to the bottom of the issue.

Over the course of my Health Champion journey, I can point to two critical turning points that shaped my perspective on where the power resides in addressing my own health issues: overcoming infertility and conquering chronic myofascial pain.

My infertility struggle taught me about the first two bullet points above—that not all health professionals are created equal, and even the top experts often need your guidance to effectively apply their knowledge to your situation. After several failed attempts at conception with the help of a "fertility expert," I was introduced to a woman who had been through a similar struggle and had done extensive research on success rates for infertility treatments across the US. Her findings were astounding. Success rates for IVF ranged from 15 to 65 percent at different clinics across the country!

After following this woman's advice and arranging to begin an IVF procedure with one of the top experts in the field (the one with a 65 percent success rate), I felt the need to ask him the same question that my previous physician couldn't answer satisfactorily. It was just a common sense question. I wanted to know if there was any way to determine whether the embryo had trouble implanting itself into my uterus. This simple question of mine (based on observations of my own personal experience and situation) caused the doctor to pause and adjust my course of diagnosis and treatment. Because he was at the leading edge of infertility research, he was aware of a new diagnostic test that could address my question. The test results revealed that there was a problem with the embryo's ability to implant into my uterus. The issue was addressed with medication and the result was a successful IVF procedure and the birth of our first daughter.

I could not have become pregnant without the doctor's help, but the doctor couldn't have helped me unless we'd had the discussion that was initiated by my question. The doctor held the knowledge of the science, but I held the responsibility for getting the most out of his expertise—by asking questions. What I'm getting at is that we will never arrive at the best possible solutions to our health problems unless we engage with the experts on our team.

The third and fourth bullet points above—that the most valuable health professionals might be found outside the traditional medical system and that they will help you coordinate various approaches to get to the bottom of the issue—are best illustrated by my quest to conquer the chronic myofascial pain condition that plagued me for thirteen years. The search eventually led me to an Exercise Physiologist, who happens to be an Olympic weightlifter. Given her credentials, I expected to just get an exercise program from her. What I got was a problem solver who guided me through various potential approaches to address the chronic pain. After hundreds of medical visits leading nowhere, I finally had someone suggesting biochemical, nutritional, chiropractic, and physical therapy (to name a few) approaches to my problem. The Exercise Physiologist was not claiming to be an expert in these fields, but she referred me to others who were.

Finding the Right Health Professional(s): They're Not All Created Equal

I can't emphasize enough how critical it is that you search until you find the right health professional(s) to help you solve your particular health problem(s). Whether this health professional ends up being an M.D., a chiropractor, an osteopath, or an exercise physiologist, what matters most is that this person is (1) an expert in the types of health problems you are facing, and (2) a holistic problem solver who considers solutions from all perspectives, which includes bringing in or recommending other health professionals with complementary expertise as needed.

It All Starts With You

No matter what, the primary responsibility rests with you. You must begin and continue the search for the right health professionals. Ask everyone you know, ask every health professional you come into contact with, and do your research. If you're not sure how to go about doing the research, find someone who can help you. Look at your social and professional networks and don't be afraid to let them know you need help finding the right health professional for your particular issue.

When it comes to finding top-rated M.D.s, there are several places to start your search; however, it will vary significantly depending on where you live. Following is a list of places to start, once you've thoroughly explored the suggestions from your social network:

- Many metropolitan area magazines will have an annual list of "top doctors." You can search the internet for local publications on top doctors. An example of the words to enter into a Google search would be "Cincinnati best doctors list"—the top result for this search is *Cincinnati Magazine's* "best doctors 2014" list, broken down by specialty.
- "Best Doctors" is a company that offers a review of your medical case by top-rated physicians in relevant fields. Although I have not had direct experience with this organization, the concept is interesting. Some employers and health insurers offer either full or partial coverage of Best Doctors services. They operate in several countries including Canada and the US. The website is bestdoctors. com. Ask your employer if this service is available to you through your health benefits, or consider contacting Best Doctors directly to learn more about their services.
- There are sites available where you can find a doctor and

see how patients have rated him or her. Examples are HealthGrades.com (US) and RateMDs.com (Canada). I would tread carefully with these, as patient satisfaction might not correlate well with a doctor's competence. In addition, there tend to be relatively few ratings per physician, so the ratings probably don't come from a representative sample of that doctor's patient population. However, if there's nothing else to go by in your area and your social network hasn't been able to help you, by all means give these sites a try.

- Look for multidisciplinary physician practices. It's generally a good sign if a physician or a group of physicians has aligned themselves with alternative or complementary practitioners. This indicates that they recognize the value of non-M.D. practitioners, which increases the chances that they are effective problem solvers and collaborators. As a bonus, they've probably done some screening of the non-M.D. practitioners affiliated with the clinic, giving you a place to start if you're looking to expand your Health Champion team. For example, the clinic where I met my exercise physiologist, the Galea Clinic in Etobicoke, Ontario is headed up by a sports medicine doctor. There are chiropractors, physiotherapists, a naturopath, a nutritionist, and a massage therapist among other practitioners affiliated with the clinic. Everyone communicates and collaborates around individual patient issues. When I meet anyone with a problem that appears to be musculoskeletal in nature (muscle, connective tissue, bones, and joints) including chronic pain, I direct them to one of the practitioners within that clinic. In fact, I have received feedback from at least three friends to date who have been helped immensely by one practitioner or another at the Galea Clinic.

Look for Evidence of Experience and Success Rates

As I mentioned previously, the evidence of success rates between infertility clinics is publicly available information on the Centers for Disease Control (CDC) website. Once I drew upon my social network and discovered this fact, it was an eye-opener. I was shocked to see the range in success rates between clinics. Even today, with all the progress made in this area, the national US average for pregnancy rate per embryo transfer for women aged thirty-five to thirty-seven is 37.8 percent compared with 57.4 percent for the Colorado Center for Reproductive Medicine, where both my daughters were conceived. And if the average rate is 37.8 percent, you know there are many clinics with a success rate much lower than 37.8 percent for that age group! If you or anyone you know is dealing with infertility, you need to check out this site: cdc.gov/art/index.htm.

Keep in mind that publicly available information about quality of medical procedures varies by country and by medical condition. To the best of my knowledge, for example, there is no publicly available data for IVF success rates by clinic in Canada. There is some information, however, regarding the average success rate in Canada.[17]

You are much more likely to find objective quality-related information at the practitioner or clinic level in the US. However, if you can't find hard data for a particular health professional, you need to go back to asking questions and assessing the quality of the responses you're getting. Challenge the doctor or clinic to provide you with hard numbers (percentage success rates) and ask for an explanation on how these compare to the national average. Their willingness to answer you directly should tell you something. If they do provide you with numbers, bear

---

[17]ivf.ca/article/statistics/human-assisted-reproduction-live-birth-rates-canada

in mind that these are unaudited. However, it is certainly better than going in blind.

Tips for Evaluating Potential Team Members

When assessing the relative value of a particular health professional, there are typically five scenarios that should raise red flags for you. Have you been consistently faced with one or more of the following responses by your health professional when describing your problem and/or sharing your hypotheses?

1. "Stop Doing That."

Remember the joke where the patient says, "Doctor, it hurts when I do this," and the doctor says, "Then don't do that."? The sad thing is that this actually happens every day in real patient/doctor interactions. In fact, it happens so frequently that I thought it useful to share several examples from my own experience and those of many others with whom I've had discussions on the topic.

1. In 2012, I experienced episodes of chest pain, nausea, and other concerning symptoms that led me to the emergency room at my nearby hospital. A quick assessment by the ER physician indicated I might have a condition called pericarditis, which is inflammation of the lining of the heart. In a follow–up consultation with a disinterested cardiologist, I was told that I likely did not have pericarditis. When I asked about what might have caused my symptoms and how to handle triathlon training, he answered, "Just don't push yourself too hard." That was it. No other explanation, no effort to uncover what was behind the symptoms. If I had listened to him, the chances of completing a half-iron triathlon in 2012 and going on to a full distance IRONMAN triathlon in 2013 would

have been slim. I might have been stuck for months, taking it easy, and worrying that I had a heart problem of some sort.

Because I didn't like what I heard and there seemed to be a gap in the information, I persevered and found another cardiologist with a problem-solving mindset. After thorough questioning about my medical and athletic history and several diagnostic tests, the doctor concluded that my symptoms were caused by a combination of low iron levels and tight chest muscles; these were resolved with iron supplements and stretching of my chest muscles, especially after long bike rides.

2. I met a man with a partially amputated foot who explained to his doctor that he still felt a lot of pain when he pushed down into his prosthetic. For example, it really hurt when he pushed down on the clutch of his standard car. The doctor's response was, "Just get an automatic."

3. A woman told her doctor that her eyes swelled when she applied eye makeup. The doctor's solution was, "Stop wearing eye makeup."

4. A young professional, active woman was looking for solutions to her urinary incontinence. She liked wearing form-fitting clothes, which don't lend themselves to wearing pads to absorb the leaks. Her doctor came back with the flip response, "Just wear looser clothes."

These doctors were completely missing the point by ignoring each patient's individual definition of quality of life. The patient wants the problem solved in order to continue doing what he/she wants with his/her life, while the doctor just wants to put a band-aid on the problem and get the patient out of the office as quickly as possible. If you can't get your doctor past this type of mindset, then you need to keep doing your research and look elsewhere for help. Don't accept a lack of clear, logical explanations and vague statements like "just stop doing that" or "don't push yourself" from health professionals.

2. "I Can't Hear You."

Some health professionals completely ignore the details you provide related to your problem. The fact that my mother dropped a couch on her big toe should have been a significant clue to the problem with her toe. Instead, because he saw an inflamed big toe in an elderly woman, the doctor chose to ignore her input and hypothesized that she had gout. As a result, he ordered unnecessary blood tests to rule out gout. I'll give you three guesses as to the result of the blood tests!

I went to my family doctor with a persistent red eye. He suspected allergies. I indicated to him that I've had allergies my entire life, and that this eye redness was not due to allergies; it was different. He insisted I apply allergy drops into the eye, and that I come back to see him if the redness didn't go away. I went back to him two more times before he finally referred me to an ophthalmologist who immediately identified a condition requiring anti-inflammatory drops.

Imagine the inefficiencies in our healthcare system arising from these types of one-sided interactions between physician and patient. If you are faced with this blatant disregard for your description of the circumstances surrounding your problem, it should be a warning signal that this physician or health professional is not the problem solver you're looking for.

In certain cases, however, a good health professional might explain to you why your description of the circumstances may not be related to a suspected problem. This was the case in 2003, when I developed severe back pain—yet another acute injury stemming from having weak and stiff muscles. An orthopedic surgeon diagnosed me with a herniated disc, but he made it clear that this problem was not the cause of my generalized chronic pain symptoms, as I had been hypothesizing. He explained that there was another underlying problem that needed to be addressed. Although he didn't know what the underlying problem was, he clearly explained which symptoms were related to the herniated disc and which were not. I didn't get the answers I wanted on the spot, but this was a useful interaction that helped me move forward in my continued search for answers to the underlying chronic pain problem.

3. "How Quickly Can I Get You out of Here?"

Sadly this is the feeling we commonly get during a typical interaction with a physician (and sometimes with other health professionals). The fact is the more patients they see in one day, the more money they make. However, there is a difference between someone working efficiently and giving you helpful direction in the shortest amount of time possible and someone who clearly wants to gloss over the problem and get you out, regardless of whether they've addressed your health objectives or not. If you leave each visit feeling like you were rushed out before you could even communicate your objectives, you might want to start looking around.

I have found that I can extend my welcome in a high-speed physician's office by being well-prepared with research and a logical line of questioning in hand. Because things can happen so fast with these types of practitioners, it's best to have your facts and questions written down in advance and readily available as you walk into the examining room.

And for any health professional who charges you directly for services, watch out for what seem to be "piecemeal" service charges. The chiropractor I saw before meeting Dr. Carm Stillo was charging me a full fee for each type of treatment he provided. For example, it was $85 for acupuncture and $85 for Active Release Therapy (ART); I had to choose which treatment I was getting that day. Carm, on the other hand, charges me one fee per visit, and I receive whatever treatment(s) I need during that visit.

4. "It Must Be in Your Head."

In some cases, the health professional might actually listen to your symptom description and do some diagnostic tests that turn out to be negative. And despite your continued complaints about your symptoms, he or she might try to convince you there's nothing wrong with you (thus implying it's all in your head). Trust your instincts. Symptoms are real if you feel them, and you need to keep searching for the cause until you get to the bottom of them. Don't let anyone tell you there's nothing wrong because they can't come up with a positive test result.

If I hear one more story about someone being told by their doctor that there is nothing wrong with them, despite clearly articulated symptoms, I'm going to scream! I recently met a woman who told me about her excruciating headaches that continued for months after having recovered from a broken jaw. She was in so much pain that she would vomit almost every day, especially when exposed to bright light. The neurologist she saw admonished her for wasting his time, as he was busy with "patients who really needed his help." Whatever tests he had conducted showed no concrete cause for the symptoms this woman described, so his approach was to completely ignore her plea for relief from the unbearable pain.

Luckily, this woman was directed to a naturopath who, after one visit, determined that it was a nerve problem and used manual therapy to give her unimaginable relief from her horrific pain. So if you have real symptoms, DO NOT STOP looking for help, no matter what doctors and other health professionals are telling you. Do your own research and ask a lot of questions of many different health professionals. There is help out there, but it's not always in the most obvious places.

5. "Don't Fill Your Head With All That Information."

If you consistently get this type of response when presenting your questions and hypotheses based on your research, this health professional shouldn't be included in your team of problem solvers. Health professionals with the right knowledge and the inclination to problem solve should be able to clearly and respectfully address any questions or hypotheses you present to them whether they agree or disagree with the information.

When I presented my understanding of pericarditis to the cardiologist who was unwilling to help me solve my problem (example from #1 above), he told me to stop reading "all that stuff on the internet." Knowledgeable problem solvers, like the second cardiologist who uncovered the issues behind my symptoms, will take your input into account and consider all solutions to the problem. Then they will explain their rationale for the diagnosis and address whether and how your research findings might fit into the picture. If they believe you're way off base with your internet research, all they have to do is let you know why.

Also watch out for health professionals who keep you coming back repeatedly for the same treatments when you're seeing no improvements. If a practitioner is getting paid for every visit, you need to know upfront how many visits are necessary before you can assess the effectiveness of the treatments. If you can't engage them in a conversation around why the treatment might not be working and what alternatives exist, it's probably a red flag indicating the need to look for a replacement for this team member.

Ask yourself if the health professionals you've met so far have been prepared to partner with you in your quest to get to the bottom of your health problem. If you can identify and have access to top experts in the field, insist on seeing them early in the process. This might mean you have to work on convincing the "gatekeepers" that you need to see the experts. In North America, the gatekeepers are often the general practitioners or family physicians.

Thinking Outside the Box to Broaden Your Team

How much investigating have you done outside the M.D.-driven medical system? What other types of health professionals might have the expertise to help you? As is the case with identifying M.D.s, make sure you inquire within your social network to see if anyone with a similar condition to yours has had success with a particular alternative practitioner. And as I mentioned earlier, multidisciplinary clinics are also good places to start when it comes to identifying qualified alternative practitioners. From my experience, I've learned that it's better to start with practitioners other than M.D.s if the problem is mainly in the soft tissues (muscles, connective tissues) and/or if your main complaint is generalized stiffness and pain that is difficult to link to a specific event. I've had significant help from various types of practitioners, some of whom I list below. Because exercise physiologists and structural integrationists are a little more difficult to find, I've given you some references to the organizations that certify or accredit them so that you can contact them either online or by phone to find a professional in your area:

- Certified or Registered Exercise Physiologist. These practitioners will generally have a Master's degree in kinesiology or exercise physiology. You can begin by identifying a qualified person by searching the following sites. In Canada, certification rests with the Canadian Society for Exercise Physiology: csepmembers.ca/english/search.asp. In the US, there is accreditation under the American College of Sports Medicine: members.acsm.org/source/custom/ Online_locator/OnlineLocator.cfm (choose "Registered Clinical Exercise Physiologist" from the Certification/ Registry Level menu).

- Clinical or Holistic Nutritionist
- Chiropractor
- Naturopath
- Osteopath/Osteopathic massage therapist
- Pilates Instructor
- Structural Integrationist (registered massage therapist with significant additional training in the Rolf Method of Structural Integration). I recommend ensuring the individual is certified by doing a search on the Rolf Institute website: rolf.org.
- Yoga Instructor

Following is a list of other types of non-M.D. practitioners you might want to look into, depending on the type of health challenges you're facing:

- Acupuncturist
- Ayurvedic Medicine Practitioner
- Homeopath
- Nurse Practitioner
- Occupational Therapist
- Pharmacist
- Traditional Chinese Medicine Practitioner

You need to do your homework and assess whether or not these practitioners are high performers, team players, and natural problem solvers, as is the case with anyone you consider adding to your Health Champion team. Once you've identified a practitioner, find out about their clientele and their personal background. As an example, my exercise physiologist, chiropractor, and nutritionist are in high demand by professional and Olympic athletes. The structural integrationist who worked on me did his clinical training while recovering from a cycling accident, after developing chronic myofascial pain. When I described my symptoms, he knew what I was talking about from personal experience.

Further, you might want to consider looking for a health coach or someone who specializes in guiding others through the process of solving healthcare challenges. This could significantly speed up the process of finding the right health professionals to help you solve your specific problem.

My Thoughts on General Practitioners and Specialists

One of my first jobs out of school was as a pharmaceutical sales representative. Through my interaction with many physicians, both general practitioners and specialists, I soon realized how broad was the spectrum of talent and motivation levels between individual physicians. I remember thinking to myself, "I would only feel comfortable sending family members to about five percent of the doctors with whom I'm interacting!"

Despite the many differences between the medical systems in the United States and Canada, there are significant similarities beginning with the process of driving patients to a primary care provider like a General Practitioner (GP) first for "triage" of various health problems. Essentially, the GP assesses the problem, determines if he/she can handle it, or whether the patient needs to be referred elsewhere for diagnosis or treatment. In theory, this should work. However, GPs face incredible time pressures as they try to see as many patients per day as possible in order to make a reasonable salary. This is not necessarily the doctors' fault, but rather is a problem with the method by which doctors are paid. In the majority of cases, they are incentivized to plow through as many cases as possible per day, which doesn't leave much time for listening to a patient's full story about their condition. Nor does it allow the physician the proper time needed to thoroughly think through all the "clues" presented by the patient in order to solve the problem holistically.

The fact that the physician is usually pressed for time reinforces the need for patients to come to their doctor's appointment well prepared and able to succinctly describe the history and symptoms of their problem. I would also encourage you to have some hypotheses about what the problem might be, based on your research. If you present your doctor with a "best guess" diagnosis, it will at least initiate a conversation about why he/she does or does not agree with your best guess. Don't be afraid to ask a lot of questions. If you're not getting satisfactory answers or the solutions offered by your GP are not working, don't hesitate to request a referral to a specialist.

The other challenge facing us when visiting a GP is the fact that they are often not well versed in alternative approaches to healthcare. Because the general mentality of Western doctors is that they hold the answers to most health issues, they often don't think "outside the box" or encourage patients to seek alternative solutions. And they tend to look at the presenting health issue without considering what's happening with the whole patient. Most chronic or complex health problems are multifaceted and vary by individual patient. As Dr. Manon Bolliger, N.D. puts it, "Treating a 'disease' without treating the person who developed it is pointless." So many times during my thirteen-year struggle, I showed up at my GP's office with one soft tissue injury after another. Every time, he or she would address the immediate injury without considering what might be behind the unending parade of injuries that plagued me. But because I was unconsciously handing over the problem-solving power to the physicians, I didn't think to prompt them to look at my problem in a more holistic way.

As is the case with GPs, there is a wide disparity between the worst and the best specialist in any discipline. Although there is a higher probability of the specialist being able to diagnose your problem, that doesn't necessarily mean that they will get it right. Remember the clueless cardiologist who couldn't tell me what my symptoms meant? In addition, I consulted at least seven different specialists in the early days of my myofascial pain syndrome, with no success.

From my observations, I've concluded that specialists are trained to look for signs of diseases and conditions that fit within their particular specialty area. The assumption is that the GP referring you has done a good job of categorizing your symptoms and that your issues will fit into the specialist's area. For example, my myofascial symptoms could be consistent with some arthritic conditions or something that might fit within a rheumatologist's realm of knowledge. The rheumatologists I saw looked for specific conditions that might be associated with my symptoms. Once the examinations and blood tests came back negative, ruling out their hypotheses, I was given a prescription for anti-inflammatories and sent home reassured that there was nothing wrong with me. This is where I failed myself. By accepting their conclusions, I internalized the fact that there were likely no solutions to my condition. After all, the specialists couldn't find anything. This significantly stymied my search for answers. Don't accept someone telling you that you're fine because they can't find any concrete evidence of a textbook condition. Not only do you need to keep looking for the right specialists within the M.D. community, but you also need to go deeper and reach out to practitioners such as naturopaths, osteopaths, or chiropractors, depending on your specific problem.

Making the Most of Every Interaction

If you choose to not deal with an issue, then you give up your right of control over the issue and it will select the path of least resistance.
Susan Del Gatto

Have you effectively communicated to your health professionals the impact of your condition on the quality of your life? Have you researched information about your symptoms, and formulated one or two hypotheses regarding what might be going on? This is not intended for you to self-diagnose, but rather to get the conversation started with your health professional. Give them something to respond to. This will allow you to evaluate their response, and it can also stimulate their thinking related to additional approaches to your particular problem. Don't be afraid to ask multiple questions during visits with health professionals. Be curious. You'd be amazed where this can lead.

The following websites are good places to start for conducting a search in preparation for your medical appointments:

- mayoclinic.org
- WebMD.com
- nlm.nih.gov/medlineplus

Note that these are mainstream health information sources. I use these when trying to come up with a hypothesis to a health problem that is likely not musculoskeletal. If your problem is musculoskeletal, it is difficult to find a trustworthy site with high quality information online. Your best bet is to try and find a good multidisciplinary sports medicine clinic and start with a sports medicine doctor or other practitioner affiliated with that clinic.

What I mean by doing research and formulating a hypothesis

around your health problem is to go through a specific thought and research process, with the goal of effectively communicating your symptoms and the circumstances surrounding them. If possible, present your best guess of what's going on as a way of initiating the dialogue with your health professional. I'm talking about a pretty straightforward process, which you can probably get through in fifteen minutes or less. The longer you've been dealing with the issue without resolution, the more time you should be spending on the research phase of the process, in order to trigger further analysis by health professionals.

Let's go through a hypothetical example. You notice a rash on your leg, which has been there for several days now, so you want to have it checked out by a doctor:

1. Write down when you first noticed the symptom(s)—in this case, the rash. Be as specific as you can by looking at your calendar and recalling each day so you can pinpoint the first time you noticed it.
2. Think about the circumstances around the time you first noticed the symptoms. Write down everything you can think of that might be relevant in helping the doctor solve the problem.
   a. What were you doing? Were you using any new products, wearing new clothes, doing anything that involved the possibility of something unusual contacting your skin? This seemingly minor detail can really help the doctor narrow the possibilities in the problem-solving process. If you're sure there was nothing of this nature, that's also very valuable information.
   b. Did you try any new foods around the time you started to notice the rash?
   c. Did you go anywhere unusual around that time?

3. Go to a reliable website like mayoclinic.org and conduct a search based on the symptoms you're experiencing and any surrounding circumstances you came up with. For example, let's say you can't identify anything that might be linked to the start of the rash. In the search bar at the top of the Mayo Clinic website, I entered the general search terms, "skin rash." This showed me a menu of choices related to skin rashes. I selected "skin rashes that itch" and this pulled up a twelve-slide presentation with pictures of the twelve most common types of skin rashes. You could look through and identify whether any of the rash patterns resemble yours.

4. Bring the information (either the image or just the name of the rash you identified) to your doctor's appointment, along with the details on when it started and any surrounding circumstances (whether you think they're relevant or not).

5. Start the conversation with your doctor by describing the symptoms and when they started. Then add whatever details you can remember about the surrounding circumstances. Depending on whether or not you're satisfied with your doctor's explanation of what type of rash it could be and his/her recommendations for diagnostics or treatment approaches, you can present your thoughts on what you found on the Mayo Clinic website. Probe into your doctor's opinion about the information you found.

If the situation is one in which you've been dealing with a known condition for some time (instead of a new, unknown problem as described in the example above), then your preparation would be different. Your research would be centered around your specific condition, and possibly some different types of interventions that could further improve your symptoms.

Let's say you have been told you have high blood pressure and you've been prescribed a medication for it. You have a follow-up appointment with your doctor and you want to know if the medication alone is enough or if there's more you can do to reduce your health risks caused by high blood pressure. Here's my recommendation on how to proceed:

1. Go to a credible website (I'll use WebMD.com this time) and simply start with the search terms "high blood pressure." The top search result is "Hypertension/High Blood Pressure Health Center." Under that title are several sub-topics, one of which is "Treatment and Care." That looks relevant, so click on that one. In this section, you'll find a large amount of information, organized in sub-sections. I clicked on "Complementary and Alternative Treatment for Hypertension" and found a very good list of options and their relative value for helping to control blood pressure. You can select one or two approaches that appear to be effective, and are of interest to you—for example, practicing yoga.

2. In your follow-up appointment with your doctor, bring up the fact that you were looking up other things you could do to bring down your blood pressure, and that you're thinking about starting a regular yoga practice. How does your doctor react? Is he/she engaged and encouraging? Is he/she offering additional non-drug suggestions? This provides you with another opportunity to assess the value of this health professional as a team member.

3. If your doctor doesn't give you a compelling reason for avoiding yoga (and if he/she does, you need to probe into why), your next step could be to begin looking for a well-established yoga studio. See my suggestions in Chapter 10 related to finding a good yoga studio and instructor.

Questions Can Lead to Productive Interactions

Many missed clues on the part of both my mom and her health professionals led to her losing most of the vision in one eye due to macular degeneration. The good news is that once this was identified and diagnosed, she was referred to a very knowledgeable ophthalmologist who provided her with the treatments needed to preserve what little sight she had remaining in the damaged eye. More importantly, having him as a resource was going to be critical for protecting the vision in her good eye. After doing some of my own research on macular degeneration, I asked to come along on one of her follow-up visits with this specialist. My goal was to make sure my mom had all the information and guidance necessary to prevent the loss of vision in her good eye.

During the doctor's visit, I could tell he was an expert in his field by the way he answered my questions directly and without hesitation or condescension. One of my questions pertained to the usefulness of low-dose aspirin in reducing the risk of macular degeneration, as it had come up in my research. He responded that the data was not supportive of this; however, he added, "Oh, yes, that reminds me. Your mom should make sure she takes omega-3 supplements, since there is some good evidence that those are protective to the eyes."

The lesson in this case is that asking a question, any question, can lead to more solutions. There are no bad questions if you are dealing with a knowledgeable health professional. It's about initiating a dialogue that can trigger further problem-solving by your health professional. You are ultimately responsible for solving your own health problems; health professionals are just one of your resources on this problem-solving journey.

I encourage you to keep researching and learning more about your condition. I'm always surprised by how much new information I find every time I conduct a new search. And this process provides fodder for further questions to trigger a productive dialogue with the right health professionals.

Request to Know All Your Options

Also, make sure you push your health professional to present *all* the treatment options so that you can make the choice that will work best for your lifestyle. Physicians might steer you toward the treatment that has the best efficacy on paper, but what if it's a treatment that you can't tolerate?

For several years, Rod had been telling me that I snored a lot and actually woke myself up frequently throughout the night—symptoms of possibly having sleep apnea. In 2011, I came across information that linked the lack of quality sleep to fibromyalgia symptoms. Knowing that fibromyalgia symptoms are very similar to those of my myofascial pain syndrome, I wondered whether there would be a link in my case. So I decided to bring up the snoring problem with my family doctor who referred me to a sleep specialist. This doctor really knew his data regarding sleep apnea, a condition in which the patient stops breathing in the middle of the night. He answered all my questions confidently, quoted the literature, and appreciated the fact that I had done my research in advance. I respected his opinion. His recommendation was a sleep study in which they would evaluate whether or not my snoring was related to apnea and if so, how serious the apnea was. To my surprise, the sleep study revealed that I stopped breathing over 150 times during the night, indicating that I had moderate to severe sleep apnea. I also learned that, if left untreated, sleep apnea is associated with a much higher risk of heart disease and a shortened life expectancy. Could this be yet another piece of the puzzle related to my myofascial symptoms? Whether it was or not, I needed to deal with this apnea.

The sleep specialist informed me that the most effective

treatment for sleep apnea is a CPAP (Continuous Positive Airway Pressure) machine. It is 95 percent effective in reducing apneic episodes. This sounded great. But as I sat with the CPAP consultant, my heart sank. In fact, I felt a lump in my throat and almost started crying. They expected me to wear a mask attached to a tube leading to a machine that would force air into my mouth and nose all night. It sounded like Darth Vader would be in the room. After almost twenty years of marriage, I wasn't overly concerned about looking unsexy to my husband, but still ... I had a little bit of vanity left in me. I had to go away and think about it. Rod and I talked about it, and the conclusion was that I needed to get the machine, which I reluctantly picked up soon thereafter.

It was a mental, emotional, and physical struggle to try to keep the mask on every night. I could not figure out how anyone could use this machine every night for the rest of their lives. Not only did I feel confined and claustrophobic when putting the mask on, making it difficult to get to sleep, but I would also unconsciously remove the mask in the middle of the night. I wasn't sure for how many hours I actually wore it. Apparently, there isn't much benefit in wearing the mask for less than five hours. According to some reports, between 60 and 90 percent of CPAP users stop using their machines by the end of the first year. This was no surprise to me, given my experience with it. What good is 95 percent efficacy if you don't actually use the treatment?

After struggling with the CPAP machine for about three months, I started to search for an alternative. I consulted a lot of people including health professionals and did some internet searches. Finally, I came upon a solution that might work. It was a custom molded dental appliance that keeps the jaw in a position that reduces the likelihood of the throat closing. The sleep specialist indicated that the effectiveness of these appliances was only around 75 percent, so he did not recommend them to his patients.

As much as I respected his knowledge, I had to separate the science from the real life application of his recommended solution. By my calculations, 95 percent effectiveness applied zero percent of the time equals zero effectiveness. By contrast, if I achieved 75 percent effectiveness applied 100 percent of the time by wearing the dental appliance nightly, I was achieving 75 percent effectiveness. Pretty simple math. So I proceeded with a consultation on a dental appliance.

Then I was faced with a tough financial decision. While the CPAP machine was fully paid for by the government health program, this dental appliance would cost me $2,300 and there was no reimbursement available from either the government or our employers' health plans. Once again, Rod's calm and rational approach encouraged me to invest in my health, quality of life, and longevity. We would find the $2,300. In the grand scheme of things, it really wasn't that much money to treat a condition that we knew was not only reducing my quality of life, but also putting my life at risk.

To this day, I use my dental appliance about 98 percent of the time, which by my calculations gives me a 70 percent reduction in apneic episodes. This is perfectly acceptable to me. Dealing with my apnea reminded me that while health professionals are there to provide information and guidance, ultimately we must make our own educated decisions regarding our health. And asking for all the options upfront gives us the power to make the decisions that are right for us.

Remain Alert for Clues, and Share Them

My pain and stiffness would usually be worse in the week leading up to my period, and would improve with the start of my period. Also, during each of my two pregnancies, there was definitely an overall improvement in my symptoms. These are facts I should have been discussing regularly and insistently with the physicians from whom I sought help. These were clues to the systemic nature of my problem; that differences in hormone levels were impacting my symptoms. And I was the only one with that information. As mentioned previously, even the best health professionals need your collaboration and input, in order to provide you with the best care. The more clues you can identify and share with health professionals, the greater your chances of triggering their problem-solving skills. All your clues are providing a window into your individual condition. Effective problem-solving begins with a clear definition of the problem, and you are the one responsible for helping health professionals get a clear picture of your particular problem.

A Primer for Questions

Here are some starters to help you formulate questions for your interactions with health professionals:

- Can you explain why ...?
- What about ...?
- Could symptom X be related to symptom Y?
- Could symptom X be related to event Y?
- What is the purpose of ...?
- What will that (treatment, drug, exercise, etc.) do?
- What side effects should I expect with this prescription?
- What are the risks associated with this treatment?
- How long will I need to continue this treatment to see a difference?
- What are the chances for success in someone with my profile?
- Are there any other treatment options for this problem?
- What other things should I be doing to help myself?
- What do my test results show? Always follow up after test results, even if you don't get called back to the doctor's office.

- Can I get a copy of my test results?
- This test result seems very close to the top (or bottom) of the range. Could that be related in some way to my symptoms? What sort of implications could that have for my lifestyle (high level of activity, gearing up for more endurance training, trying to get pregnant, high-stress job, etc.)?
- What other tests might help us pinpoint the problem and give us more direction on finding the right solutions?

No matter how great the reputation of the health professional, ask all the questions that come to mind. The more you know about your symptoms or condition, the better your questions. And there are no bad questions. You'd be amazed at how you can trigger the professional to consider different aspects of your problem. Imagine if I hadn't asked Dr. Schoolcraft about whether the embryos could implant in my uterus.

Informed Patients Will Face Challenges ... But Don't Let That Stop You

A recent study in the *British Medical Journal* (BMJ) showed that patients who are well educated about their condition will face many challenges in gaining cooperation from physicians, nurses, and other healthcare practitioners.[18] This is something I've been encountering for a few years now, since I know more than most physicians do about chronic myofascial pain syndrome and how to effectively manage it.

In this particular study, diabetic patients were trained and challenged to think of themselves differently, as empowered and expert patients, no longer dependent on doctors for decisions, but able to talk about their treatment requirements with healthcare professionals as equals. So instead of saying things like, "My doctor told me to [take insulin at a certain time],"

---

[18] bmjopen.bmj.com/content/3/11/e003583.long

they would be encouraged to talk about the *discussions* they would be having with their doctor about how and when they should take insulin.

After receiving the training and becoming better versed than most general practitioners about their condition, the study's participants often found themselves in ambiguous roles in healthcare interactions. Many physicians and other health professionals not as knowledgeable in diabetes management did not necessarily value the informed patient's input into the treatment plan. Unfortunately, this will be an ongoing issue in our medical system until a critical mass of patients are informed enough to challenge physicians to become problem-solving partners.

On the bright side, however, if you search you can usually find a health professional who is interested in partnering with you to solve your problems; someone who respects and appreciates your knowledge if you've put in the time to do the research. Don't give up the search for the right problem-solving partner. And who knows, in the process of becoming an informed patient, you might find some answers for yourself!

Continuous Problem-Solving Is Key for Chronic Conditions

Whenever I think I've gone as far as I can with understanding and managing my chronic myofascial pain syndrome, I learn something new, which could take me to yet another level of health and physical performance. It starts with always being on the lookout for a new understanding of your condition, and anything that could be a potential solution.

In my case, I've known for several years that staying hydrated is really important to keeping the fascia (connective tissue) loose and functioning properly. My chiropractor also mentioned a few times that it's not just about drinking water.

Electrolytes are very important in ensuring adequate hydration, and some people are just naturally low in electrolytes (like me). Important electrolytes include sodium, potassium, and magnesium. I've known for four years that I tend to be low in magnesium, and so I take a daily supplement. I also drink water constantly throughout the day, and have electrolyte drinks when I'm working out.

Sometimes, you have to hear the same thing many times presented in different ways before the solution clicks. Every now and then, I do some reading on chronic myofascial pain syndrome/fibromyalgia, and look for any information I don't yet know. Once in particular, I was motivated by the pain and stiffness that began creeping back into my body with all the IRONMAN training I was doing in 2013. I came across some information that referred to injections directly into muscle tissue where there are "trigger points" (areas of contracted muscle cells that can't relax or function properly. These areas can be at least partially relieved through various techniques, including manual compression, rolling on them with a ball, acupuncture, etc.). I had made a ton of progress with all the steps I had taken to that point; however, I had not yet explored this idea of trigger-point injections.

So I booked an appointment with my sports medicine physician, Dr. Galea. His opinion was that I had too many trigger points to even begin injections. So he recommended starting with an intravenous electrolyte solution in order to fully hydrate the tissues. Then, if most trigger points responded well and subsided, we could inject any remaining stubborn ones. This made sense to me: IV electrolytes to maximize hydration of the stubborn, knotted tissue. You can get much more of the electrolytes to the tissues this way, because you're limited in how much electrolyte drink you can consume before getting nauseous. In addition to carrying electrolytes, the IV can be packed with nutrients that are known to have positive effects on myofascial tissue, like amino acids, natural anti-inflammatory agents, and antioxidants.

The four intravenous sessions had a remarkable effect on clearing up trigger points and softening up the myofascial tissue. This led to the identification of four key trigger points, which Dr. Galea injected with vitamin B12. All this happened within six weeks of the IRONMAN event, and played a signifi- cant role in my ability to show up and complete the race.

Once again, I was reminded that the answers won't be handed to me on a silver platter. There are good health professionals out there, but it's my responsibility to reach out and leverage their knowledge for my specific problem. In this example, my research triggered a question, and my question triggered a discussion. When presented with my question, the expert was challenged to think about an alternative approach to my prob- lem. This is the power of problem-solving as part of a Health Champion team.

Leave No Stone Unturned: Ask Questions About Medical Test Results

Not only is it important to research your symptoms and ask questions of your healthcare professionals to increase your chances of finding solutions, but you must also carefully review the results of any diagnostic tests that are conducted on you. We generally rely on the fact that the doctor's office will call us if there is anything "wrong" in our test results. However, I encourage you to review your own results and discuss them in depth with your physician or other healthcare professionals, regardless of whether the results are considered "abnormal" or not.

From my experience, here are two incidences of how lab results just pass as "normal" when in fact there could be some valuable information being overlooked by not paying more at- tention to the details.

On the advice of my exercise physiologist in 2009, I had a thorough blood analysis done, to see whether nutrient and/or hormone deficiencies might be contributing to my chronic pain and stiffness. She noted that magnesium was a mineral that was important for proper muscle contraction and relaxation, and it would be interesting to see what my level was. So I requested the blood test from my sports medicine doctor and booked an appointment to review the results.

The magnesium test showed a level of 0.71 mmol/L, with a "reference" range of 0.70-1.00 mmol/L. Because my number fell within the reference range, it did not get flagged and my doctor would not have normally reviewed it with me. However, because of what I learned about magnesium and muscle function, I wanted to talk about this. Based on our discussion, he agreed it might help to take magnesium supplements, and he recommended supplements that contained both magnesium and calcium, as these minerals work together to regulate muscle contraction and relaxation. About three weeks after I started taking the supplements, I began feeling a significant difference. This was one of the many important pieces to my chronic pain puzzle. Without my request for the test and for a review of the results, the information would have passed unnoticed and remained filed away in my medical record.

The second incident happened in 2011, when I was well on my way to overcoming the chronic muscle stiffness, and participating in several triathlons—I almost passed out at the end of my longest race that season. My blood pressure plummeted, and I had to be treated by the paramedics on site. This was a scary experience to say the least.

When I spoke to my family doctor about the episode, she just attributed it to possible dehydration or not enough electrolytes that day, and sent me on my way because my blood pressure was perfectly normal the day I went to see her. This didn't seem right to me, so I took the question to my sports medicine doctor, who went back into my chart to look at my level of iron stores. The test (which had been done several months earlier) revealed a ferritin level of 16 ug/L. This was within the reference range of 10 ug/L to 291 ug/L. What this lab report didn't highlight was that anything below 30 ug/L indicated "depleted iron stores." In fact the "normal" level of iron stores is between 80 and 300 ug/L! For someone training to do endurance events, depleted iron stores would soon become iron deficiency, resulting in not enough oxygen available to meet the needs of the body. Again, this blood result passed through the doctor's office without a second look, because the result was not flagged as "abnormal" by the lab. It was up to me to pursue a solution to my problem.

Based on my experience and the pervasiveness of chronic pain disorders like fibromyalgia, I'm curious to know how many of us are walking around with sub-optimal levels of key minerals in our bodies. Here is a glimpse into the important functions of minerals:[19]

- **Calcium** helps build and maintain strong bones and teeth. It also helps muscles work and supports cell communication.
- **Chromium** helps maintain normal blood sugar (glucose) levels.
- **Copper** helps break down iron, helps make red blood cells, and helps produce energy for cells.
- **Iodine** works to make thyroid hormones.
- **Iron** carries oxygen to all parts of the body through red blood cells.
- **Magnesium** helps muscles and nerves work, steadies heart rhythm, maintains bone strength, and helps the body create energy.

---

[19]webmd.com/vitamins-and-supplements/minerals-and-their-functions-and-sources

- **Manganese** supports bone formation and wound healing, and also helps break down proteins, cholesterol, and carbohydrates. It's also an antioxidant.
- **Potassium** helps the nervous system and muscles, and helps maintain a healthy balance of water.
- **Selenium** helps protect cells from damage and regulates thyroid hormone.
- **Zinc** supports immune function, as well as the reproductive and nervous systems.

Minerals are obviously important to almost all our vital functions. The problem is that, although the labs have "reference" ranges for "acceptable" blood levels of these minerals in the general population, no one knows what the appropriate levels are for each individual's body to function at its optimal level. And for each individual, the minimum acceptable levels can be different, depending on one's level of activity among many other factors.

What's more is that "reference" levels from the population reflect a North American population that is depleted in minerals! In Chapter 10, I provide a comprehensive overview of why and how modern day humans have become depleted of minerals.

No matter what you're being tested for, request a copy of your test results and discuss anything that looks like it's at the bottom or top end of the "reference range" with your doctor or other health professionals. Find out if, for your lifestyle, there is any possibility that you could benefit from a higher or lower level on that particular test, and whether there are ways to achieve this. And as always, don't hesitate to take these results to another healthcare professional who specializes in the field related to the test result in question.

No matter what type of health professional you're working with, explore questions around nutritional requirements and blood analysis to determine whether there is a deficiency in elements important to addressing your problem. For most of my twenties and early thirties, I was a vegetarian who didn't like fish, eggs, or vegetables. In addition, I had lactose intolerance and avoided most dairy products. How much protein and other nutrients critical to muscle and connective tissue function do you think I was taking in on a daily basis? My diet high in inflammatory foods and low in protein and key nutrients for soft tissue function would have been bad enough for the average person, but for someone like me with an underlying soft tissue disorder, it proved disastrous. Not one doctor in my thirteen-year struggle asked me any details about my diet. If you don't bring it up, they often won't ask.

I've covered a lot of ground related to selecting the appropriate health professionals and looking for problem solvers with whom to build your Health Champion team. I've also presented many suggestions for making the most of every interaction you have with a health professional. Now it's up to you. What steps will you take to implement the information from this chapter?

For more resources, recommendations, and tips related to selecting and challenging the right health professionals, refer to the workbooks available on my website: carolestaveley.com.

Six

Step 6: Budget for Your Healthcare

Don't tell me what you value. Show me your budget, and I'll tell you what you value.
US Vice President, Joe Biden

Being a Health Champion means you are your own Chief Problem Solver. It is likely that you'll need to invest some financial resources in your health in order to get the best results possible. The amount you will need could be anywhere from negligible to astounding, but it's better to be prepared than disappointed when you come across a potential health solution that requires funding.

Like many North Americans, I believed that the only professionals qualified to treat health problems are doctors (M.D.s). Being Canadian, I assumed that our publicly funded healthcare system only pays for effective treatments. Therefore, chiropractors, osteopaths, massage therapists, yoga instructors, exercise physiologists, etc. must not provide effective solutions, since our system doesn't pay for them. Right?

My seventeen-year journey through the healthcare system, searching for an answer to my musculoskeletal problem, certainly proved that concept wrong. While our medical system has provided us with incredible improvements in longevity and quality of life, there are many aspects of health that it does not address appropriately. While doctors have a lot of knowledge, they cannot be expected to know everything. As I emphasized in Chapter 5, it is our responsibility to guide them in helping us with our particular issues. But in many cases, finding and putting together all the pieces of our health puzzle mean going beyond what's typically recognized and paid for by governments and insurance companies.

Almost all of the people, products, and services that essentially gave me my life back are not covered by our public healthcare system. And most are not even covered by private health plans. That needs to change, but that discussion is for another day. Right now, I want to discuss the importance of looking at our wellbeing as an investment. Many knowledgeable professionals and effective therapies are not recognized or paid for by public or private health insurers. Therefore, it is our own responsibility to seek them out and find a way to pay for them. You might balk at paying $90 for one session with a chiropractor, but what if he/she can really help you? What if all you needed were three sessions with a really good chiropractor to propel you to a new level of physical wellbeing? What if $200 for blood tests not covered by a health plan and $500 for a comprehensive, customized meal and supplements plan could help get you from debilitated to functional? What is that sense of physical freedom worth?

One day in 2012, I called to touch base with my brother Jehan, and he told me that he was suffering from a really sore back after lifting a heavy object. In fact, it was so sore that he was staying home from work that day. Being on contract, he was not getting paid for this sick day; this told me that he was in a lot of pain and discomfort. I asked what steps he had taken so far to try and resolve it. When the injury happened, he went to a walk-in clinic and got prescriptions for anti-inflammatories and physiotherapy; he had already completed a few sessions of physiotherapy with no improvement. In fact, he felt like it was getting progressively worse.

Based on my experience with musculoskeletal issues, I convinced him that he needed to see someone who specializes in this type of problem. I had an appointment booked with my chiropractor, Carm, that day and offered it to Jehan. He doesn't have a car, so I suggested he rent a car for the day. When he presented his symptoms and the history of how the injury occurred, Carm knew exactly what the problem was. After one treatment, Jehan told me he felt 50 percent better and dubbed Carm "The Magician." Jehan received some specific exercises to do at home, and Carm recommended one or two more visits for chiropractic treatment. In one day, Jehan was back to functioning well enough to work and carry on with activities of daily living. Within two weeks he was back to 100 percent. Jehan also learned that the exercises recommended by the particular physiotherapist he had seen were exactly the opposite of what he needed to fix this particular problem.

Jehan had to spend a total of about $350 in car rental and chiropractor fees for three visits. Considering his suffering and unpaid time away from work while he was doing the wrong exercises, was it worth it? I'll let you answer that one for yourself.

In 2000, Rod and I had to regroup after several failed attempts at conceiving with the help of a fertility clinic in Cincinnati. Then we heard about the clinic in Denver that boasted a success rate of more than double that of our existing clinic (65 percent versus 25 percent). We were faced with IVF procedure costs that were double the Cincinnati rates, plus the airfares and accommodation costs, in order to give the Denver clinic a try. We looked at how we could come up with the funds to make this happen, which was mainly a function of putting off some vacations for the next year or two. Even if we had to find a way to borrow the money, we would have done so. No matter what the outcome of this procedure, we could not rest until we knew we had tried everything in our power to have a baby. At the time, becoming parents was our WHY.

Had we followed the advice of our local Cincinnati doctor, we would have proceeded with a $20,000 egg donor program that would have been doomed to fail, just like the other attempts with my own eggs in Cincinnati. This is because my eggs were not the problem. As you know from Chapter 5, the problem that was uncovered in Denver as a result of my engaging Dr. Schoolcraft with a key question was the inability of the embryo to implant in my uterus. So how does the $20,000 IVF procedure in Denver stack up in terms of value? How do you put a price on the birth of a beautiful baby? Please remember, though, that it wasn't just about finding Dr. Schoolcraft, spending the money, and crossing our fingers. In order to get full value from this encounter, I had to ask questions and engage Dr. Schoolcraft in problem-solving *with* me.

When I advocate budgeting and putting money aside for healthcare costs, I'm not talking about throwing money around and hoping for results outside of insured services. That's just more of the same—the blind squirrel hoping to find a nut. It's critical to follow the Health Champion process and make the most of every single interaction with health professionals, no matter who pays for their services. It just so happens that when you're paying, there's both your quality of life and your bank account at stake, rather than just your quality of life.

The key point is that you can't focus on the price. You must focus on the value of what you're getting. How valuable is a day without pain, or the ability to hold your baby without developing tendinitis? What about the ability to have a good night's sleep without the help of medication to ease the pain and discomfort, or without self-medicating with alcohol? Think of what you spend money on each month (clothes, alcohol, eating out, and entertainment) and ask yourself if these are truly necessities, or if these things could be traded in for the prospect of feeling better and accomplishing so much more in life. Investing in feeling better will likely include a financial investment, as well as an investment in time and effort on your part. The quality of the rest of your life depends on your willingness to invest in your health.

How you spend your time and money is an indicator of what

you are prioritizing in your life. Go back to your WHY. What is the value of achieving the improved health state that allows you to fulfill your life purpose? Are there things that you're doing with your time and money that are not critical to improving your quality of life? It's time to redirect those resources. In what areas could you reduce spending in order to build your Health Champion fund?

Start with the following simple exercise to determine what financial resources you might be able to redirect to start your Health Champion fund.

Monthly Expense Estimates (List Items and $)

Necessary no flexibility	Necessary some flexibility	Optional

Monthly Income after tax and deductions   __________
Total "Necessary—no flexibility"   __________
Total "Necessary—some flexibility"   __________
Total "Optional"   __________
Income minus all expenses   __________

Questions to consider:

1. Take a look at the "optional" items. Which ones are not helping you achieve your WHY? Could you give them up in favor of a dedicated health fund that could help you achieve your WHY?
2. What is your "slush fund"—the money left over after you subtract all three types of expenses? Could you commit to setting that aside for your Health Champion fund every month?
3. What steps could you take to reduce the total spent on those necessary items that have some flexibility built in? Consider putting the difference into your Health Champion fund.
4. What other savings or assets do you have? Is there any possibility of redirecting at least a portion of these toward your Health Champion fund? Depending on what you've earmarked that money for, think about whether you could enjoy your future life more with less money, but a healthier mind and body.

I encourage you to look carefully at your financial situation in order to find resources to allocate toward a healthier, more fulfilling life. However, I am not a financial advisor or expert. If you're interested in delving more into the budgeting process, following are a few resources you could use:

- I recently found an article online that provides a good twelve-step overview of the budgeting process. Following is the website for this article: moneycrashers.com/how-to-make-a-budget.
- If you like the use of technology to manage various aspects of your life, you might want to try apps like "Mint" by Intuit, which allows you to set up and track budgets, manage bill payments and debt, among other functions.[20] The best part is it's all in one place and always with you on your mobile device.

If you truly can't find any personal funds to put toward health services and/or products that are not paid for by a health plan, please refer to Chapter 5 and ensure that you are fully leveraging the health professionals and services that are covered by your government or private health plan(s).

For more resources, recommendations, and tips related to budgeting for your healthcare refer to the workbooks available on my website: carolestaveley.com.

---

[20]mint.com/

SECTION II—SUMMARY

By checking the items below, you can feel confident that you've become the Chief Problem Solver in addressing your health challenges—this means you've identified the right team members, and you know how to leverage their strengths and skills to optimize the outcome of your Health Champion journey.

Step 4: Develop and Use Your Social Support Network

☐ I have at least one or two family members or close friends whom I can count on for support, no matter what. If not, I have a plan for building a closer relationship with at least one key supporter.

☐ I am committed to spending more time with supporters and less time with naysayers in my social circle.

☐ I will share my health challenges with my broader social network and welcome any suggestions they might offer.

☐ I will take action and look into suggestions made by my social connections if I believe there is even a remote possibility they could lead to identifying further solutions to enhance my health status.

Step 5: Select and Challenge the Right Health Professionals

☐ If a health professional consistently takes any of the following five approaches in dealing with my health concerns, I will look elsewhere for advice:
    ☐ Stop doing that.
    ☐ I can't hear you.
    ☐ How quickly can I get you out of here?
    ☐ It must be in your head.
    ☐ Don't fill your head with all that information.

- [ ] I will prepare for every health appointment by doing research and formulating questions intended to initiate a discussion with the health professional.
- [ ] When I believe there is a need for specialized care, I will attempt to uncover the highest rated experts in the field, and request a referral if necessary.
- [ ] I will ask to see all my test results regardless of whether they are deemed "normal." I will inquire about any findings that are at the top or bottom of a given range.
- [ ] I will ask health professionals to elaborate on all the approaches that could help improve my condition.
- [ ] If I don't feel confident or qualified to engage in discussions with health professionals, I will enlist the help of someone in my social network or hire a health coach.

Step 6: Budget for Your Healthcare

- [ ] I am committed to establishing a Health Champion fund, from which I can draw when I identify health resources that could be beneficial but are not covered by third-party health plans.
- [ ] I have completed the exercises in Chapter 6 and identified a specific amount of money that I can set aside in a dedicated account on a regular basis.
- [ ] I will look at health expenditures in terms of the potential life value they represent, rather than the price tag associated with them.

For more resources, recommendations and tips on applying the Health Champion approach, refer to the workbooks available on my website: carolestaveley.com.

SECTION III

Persevere

As you follow your WHY, set your goals, build your Health Champion team, and begin to put the puzzle together for achieving your full potential, there will most certainly be moments when you question yourself and your ability to keep moving forward. This section is intended to provide you with some tools for persisting and persevering with your Health Champion approach to ultimately keep you advancing toward your purpose.

Seven

Step 7: Fully Implement Potential Solutions

Patience, persistence and perspiration make an unbeatable combination for success.
Napoleon Hill

When a health professional hands you a prescription or recommends certain actions for you to take, how often do you ask questions like the following:

- What exactly does that do?
- Why is it important?
- How long do I need to keep taking (or doing) this to know whether it's working?

You might think it's odd for me to put the above questions under the "Perseverance" section. However, based on personal experience, I know that we humans are much more likely to follow through with recommendations when we understand *why* the recommendations are being made. Health issues aside, I can think of a recent example of behavior change that was driven by understanding "why." When I wrote my first book, the editor had deleted one space after the period at the end of every single sentence in my manuscript. In the early 1980s, one of the cardinal rules that was driven into our brains in ninth grade typing class was the need to place two spaces after every period. So when my manuscript came back with all those spaces removed, I assumed it was a book formatting thing. So I went on my merry way, continuing to place two spaces after every

121

period in everything I wrote. Just recently, when I had a marketing consultant review a brochure I had written, he pointed out that since the advent of computers, there was no longer a need to place two spaces after each period. In other words, that convention had only been necessary because of the letter spacing challenges with manual typewriters! So I was typing in a way that was obsolete. And that's all it took. That very same day, I began changing a typing style I had been implementing for more than thirty years.

When we understand what impact a recommendation can have on our condition, and what timeframe is required to fully appreciate that impact, the motivation to persevere is ignited. This time-bound link between the treatment and a desired health outcome makes it straightforward for the mind to accept. Have you ever been told to take a certain medicine on an empty stomach or with food? Have you ever asked why that's necessary? I was given a prescription once that came with instructions to take it on an empty stomach. Not knowing why that was necessary, I ignored the directions. I received no benefit from taking the medicine. In a follow-up discussion with the pharmacist, I learned that the medication is not absorbed by the body when taken within thirty minutes of eating or drinking anything other than water. I think I might have behaved differently had I been given that information in the first place.

What if I Don't Like the Recommendation?

In many cases, the recommendation might be unpleasant or uncomfortable. For example, I really hate swallowing pills to the point where I feel like I'm gagging on them. But once I understood the details behind how and why certain supplements could improve my condition if I persevered with them for several months, I had no problem forcing myself to keep taking them. Prior to understanding, I would dabble here and there with a few supplements and give up because of the unpleasantness of swallowing the pills. I now take approximately fifteen to twenty tablets and/or capsules per day. I still hate taking them, but the knowledge that they are linked to my healthier, more productive and happier life makes it a no-brainer.

Another great example from my Health Champion journey was the importance of implementing my strength training program exactly as directed by Jillian, my exercise physiologist. In fact, this was one of the mental breakthroughs that changed the course of my life. As I was "diligently" doing the exercise program that Jillian had developed for me, I found that some of the exercises were just too difficult and "didn't feel good," so I would often skip those particular exercises. Luckily, Rod also had an exercise program from Jillian that included some of these more difficult and uncomfortable exercises.

One day, as we were doing our workout program together, Rod said "those @#!* squat walks with the rubber band around the ankles are really hard, and they feel horrible."

I totally agreed with him, briefly feeling justified in skipping them altogether. But then he surprised me by saying, "I guess that's why we need to keep doing them!"

It hit me like a ton of bricks ... OF COURSE! The exercises are hard because the muscles being worked are weak and need strengthening! Looking back, it seems such common sense. However, our bodies are programmed to take the path of least resistance, so sometimes we have to tell the body to "suck it up" in order get the results we're looking for. From that point forward, I did all the exercises in my program without exception, realizing that the hardest ones (that made me swear the most) were the most important ones.

The following story from someone I recently met is probably the most powerful illustration of the point I'm trying to make in this chapter. Christine, a military nurse, suffered from post-traumatic stress disorder (PTSD) after several deployments overseas, including two in Afghanistan where she treated frontline soldiers and injured civilians. She came back from her last deployment a different person. She was depressed, negative, angry, and turning to alcohol in an attempt to erase her mental and emotional suffering. She continued searching for help, after going through several unhelpful psychiatrists, until she found someone who appeared willing to work with her to solve her problem. This psychiatrist suggested the use of Neurofeedback to essentially reprogram the way her mind was dealing with the overwhelming stress from her war experiences.

Being a nurse, Christine doubted that something as seemingly "unscientific" as Neurofeedback could have any impact on her condition. However, when she engaged the physician and asked for rationale behind the treatment, she was convinced enough to give it a try. Importantly, part of the discussion led the doctor to tell Christine she needed to give it at least six weeks before determining whether the treatment was going to provide some relief. Armed with this information, Christine was determined to follow through for at least six weeks no matter what. As it turns out, Neurofeedback was the treatment that enabled Christine to begin thinking about re-establishing her life. In her own words, it brought her "out of the basement." She gradually began to exercise again, went back to school to earn her Nurse Practitioner's degree, and celebrated her rediscovery of life by completing her first triathlon in years the summer of 2014. Which is when I had the privilege of meeting her.

If you're working with a knowledgeable health professional who is interested in helping you solve your health challenge, he/she will be more than happy to answer questions regarding the importance, relevance, and necessary timeframe of his/her recommendations. Those answers will give you confidence and motivate you to persevere. If you're not getting satisfactory answers, this might be an indication that this health professional

(1) doesn't really care about helping you solve your problem, or (2) is simply a "protocol follower" who doesn't really understand the underlying reasons for making the recommendations. In either case, this is not the health professional who can help you achieve your healthiest potential. You'll never know this unless you ask the questions and engage the health professional.

Once you understand how specific recommendations can lead you to an improved health state, be sure to follow through with one hundred percent commitment. If you don't, you're potentially missing out on an opportunity for further problem-solving. If a certain recommendation seems to be helping, keep looking for more solutions along the same lines by asking your current health professional and reaching out to others whenever possible. It's likely that the full solution involves more than one approach. Don't drop one approach in favor of another that you think might work better, at least not initially. Add the new approach to the others if at all possible. There's a good chance the benefits will be cumulative. You can later decide to try dropping one or the other to determine whether or not your improvements are sustained.

Listen closely to each health professional's point of view and pay attention to the things that provide even minor relief. These are all clues that YOU must put together to arrive at the overall solution. Pay particular attention if two or more health professionals are giving you similar advice. Keep digging for information along these lines. The more you can confirm for yourself that you're headed down the right path, the more likely you are to take action toward the recommended treatments, exercises, etc.

Don't underestimate the importance of movement, especially if your problem involves soft tissues. No matter what your condition, lack of movement will often cause more problems than it can fix. In fact, that applies to our lives in general. In his book, *What Makes Olga Run*, Bruce Grierson captures some fascinating information about the science of aging and the principles of preserving mind and body function for as long as possible. "Keep moving" is rule number one on his list, which is based on research findings and the evidence from his subject, Olga Kotelko, a ninety-three-year-old competitive track and field star. In fact, there is scientific evidence showing that even spending more time in an upright position versus sitting or lying down results in a myriad of health benefits that are linked to a longer life.[21] If you can't stand up, any kind of regular movement throughout the day is beneficial.

Remain open to accepting and implementing unfamiliar approaches. Nobel Laureate James Watson (co-discoverer of DNA) once said: "Men of fifty don't like to fail. That's why they're so dull." Trying new things can feel risky as we get older. However, fear of failure leads to half-heartedness, which in turn leads us unknowingly to forego opportunities that life has to offer.

Can you think of instances when certain treatments or approaches were recommended to you, but you didn't fully understand their purpose and, therefore, you decided to ignore them? Have any suggestions been made to you for improving your condition that you might not have fully implemented, if at all? It might be time to revisit these, ask the questions that will help you understand the recommendations and their role in your health improvement journey, then implement the ones that make sense to you.

---

[21]Joan Vernikos, Ph.D., *Sitting Kills, Moving Heals*. Quill Driver Books, 2011

Eight

Step 8: Find Everyday Motivators to Keep You Going

*Motivation is deeply personal and only you
know what words or images will resonate with
you.*
Daniel H. Pink (from his book *Drive*)

No matter how strong the emotional pull of your WHY, there will be days when you tell yourself that doing your exercises or following through on the necessary actions to improve your condition are optional. "What will it matter if I skip it today?" you might ask yourself. We all need a little extra push some days. If you're lucky, your social support network might kick in and talk you into action. However, there will be many times when you're on your own, and you'll have to answer to yourself after making the choice to do the right thing or not. On this topic, I'd like to share some approaches that work for me, as well as some suggestions from my limited yet interesting readings in behavioral psychology and related fields.

The Power of Choosing the Right Music

I have long relied on powerful and inspiring lyrics to motivate me to action and to push me to the next level. It all started with my love of a band called "The Alarm" in my university years. What I realized was that it wasn't just about the music: it was the powerful lyrics that drew me in. This band's songs almost always conveyed a message of never giving up and fighting for what you want in life. In order to use music as a propelling force in your life, not only must you enjoy the music, but the lyrics must be powerful motivators for you. And, believe it or not, it is not easy to find these types of songs. It has taken me four years to accumulate just fifty-two songs on my playlist, which I've dubbed "Believe."

Of course, I enjoy the musical arrangements, but in order for a song to make it onto the "Believe" playlist, the words have to resonate. A copy of my playlist can be found in "References and Resources" at the end of this book. Here are some examples of why I selected these artists' songs.

"Anything" by Hedley

With lyrics like "I can do anything," this song has come in handy more than once. It recently entered my mind and pushed me onward, as I was about to quit halfway through my swim practice.

"Feel This Moment" by Pitbull With Christina Aguilera

This song has a great beat, a powerful voice, and is a really good reminder that we need to "feel" every moment of our lives. Make every minute count. Don't just say it, live it. *Carpe diem.*

"The Fighter" by Gym Class Heroes

"Until the referee rings the bell ... Gonna live life till we're dead" Try giving this a listen while you work out, and see what happens to your intensity and determination!

"Inner Ninja" by Classified

"You find that extra 'uh' and push your way through it." This reminds me that I need to keep pushing through the dark times, because there is always light on the other side.

"Skyscraper" by Demi Lovato

I'm not the biggest fan of Demi Lovato's music in general, but when someone pointed out to me the lyrics of this song, I fell in love with it. If you listen for the lyrics, you can't help but feel determined and empowered! The key inspiring line for me is "I will be rising from the ground like a skyscraper." I picture talking to my physical limitations when I hear these words.

"Spirit of 76" by The Alarm

"I will never give in, until the day that I die." This one line has helped propel me through many difficult moments. When I heard those words in 2009 while trying to decide whether to show up and do my first triathlon, it strengthened my resolve to go for it, despite the many doubts in my mind about my ability to finish it.

"#thatPOWER" by Will.i.am

This is the song that made its way into my brain as I entered the water at the start of my IRONMAN event in 2013. And it stayed with me as if it were on "repeat" through the entire 14 hours and 47 minutes of the race. "Bigger, better, stronger, power. I got that power." When I play it now, it fills me with the belief that I really can do anything I set my mind to.

You can take inspiring words from any song and make them apply to your situation. Make them meaningful for you. For example, the song "Try" by Blue Rodeo is actually about a relationship, but I just hear the words, "Don't you know you have to try?" and I immediately think about overcoming my physical issues to reach my goals. So what's on *your* "Believe" playlist? It could make the difference between stagnancy and progress on the road to reaching your full potential.

The Power of Choosing the Right Images

As mentioned in Chapter 4, there is solid evidence that even the picture of someone we love and trust will cause us to be more motivated and perform at a higher level. You can strategically place photos of your supportive loved ones (both living and departed) in places you will regularly see them: the screensaver on your computer, the background on your phone, on the fridge, on your night table.

Another potent visual motivator can be an image that represents your WHY. It can even be the words you've found to verbalize your WHY, for example "Maximizing Potential" for me. They might not do much for you, but when I see those words I know what's behind them. For me, those words stand for giving my kids the best odds of success, achieving my full potential, and developing a rewarding career of helping others achieve their healthiest potential. Come to think of it, I will be prominently displaying those words wherever I can, in addition to pictures of my kids and husband.

Think about the sounds and images that trigger powerful feelings like determination and drive for you. You might need to go back many years and conjure up situations in which you felt particularly motivated and determined. What music, sounds, and images were associated with those moments? Who in your life (whether living or departed) has had a supportive and positive impact on you? Where can you post their images for maximum impact? Get creative and find ways to surround yourself with sounds and images that will trigger you to focus on your WHY and fill you with the willpower to say "no" to the gremlins of self-defeat.

Nine

Step 9: Never, Ever Give Up!

Never, Never, Never Give Up.
Attributed to Winston Churchill

One of the key factors that drove my ability to keep going over the years was a gradual understanding that nothing worthwhile in life comes easily. If I'm presented with a wonderful opportunity, it will take work, frustration, sweat, and maybe some tears to fully realize it. Once we expect challenges, difficulties, disappointments, and setbacks, they don't seem so overwhelming when they present themselves to us. According to Brené Brown, Ph.D., author of *The Gifts of Imperfection*, hope is a product of *believing in yourself, persisting,* and being able to *tolerate disappointment.* Think about that for a moment. This is based on years of social research. Not only do we need to believe in ourselves; we need to cultivate a tolerance for disappointment in order to maintain our hope for a better future. Hope is that light at the end of the tunnel that drives us to persevere. Expect disappointment, and it won't freeze you in your tracks when it smacks you in the face. You'll observe it, acknowledge it, push it aside, and continue to strive toward your WHY.

Turning Adversity Into Advantage

Dr. Paul Stoltz's research has shown that the difference between those he calls Climbers (who learn, grow, strive, and improve until their final breath), Campers (who do what it takes to get to a certain level and then settle down well below the summit), and Quitters (who simply give up on the pursuit of an enriching life and end up embittered) is what they do with adversity. In his book, *The Adversity Advantage* (Fireside, 2010), Dr. Stoltz outlines a strategy for leveraging adversity to our advantage, which includes envisioning our life on the other side of the adversity, focusing on the things we can control, and what actions we can take to minimize the downside and maximize the upside of the situation.

Dr. Stoltz wrote his book with Erik Weihenmayer, a blind man who succeeded in climbing the seven highest mountain peaks in the world. If anyone can inspire you to recognize the power of taking on adversity, it's Erik Weihenmayer. His message is that no matter how big our adversities may be, we can increase the impact and richness of our lives by facing the challenges head-on. In *The Adversity Advantage*, Erik recounts his heart-stopping adventures and gruelling challenges in preparing for and climbing the highest mountains in the world. He provides some techniques for increasing your ability to use adversity as fuel in those moments when you just want to "pull the covers over your head"—your MRI results were not good, or your tenth medical appointment revealed no new information about reducing your pain.

Aside from doing things like breaking down overwhelming tasks into small steps that can be celebrated and visualizing how it will feel to "cross the finish line," he adds a few interesting approaches like "positive pessimism," which I found intriguing and began using for myself. After Rod and I finished reading *The Adversity Advantage* in the summer of 2013, we had an opportunity to use positive pessimism when we were out on a very long bike ride as part of my IRONMAN training (Rod was also training for an endurance event). It seemed whatever direction we went, the wind was in our faces. Rod turned to me and said, "It might be all uphill, but at least it's windy!" We both laughed and felt the burning in our legs and lungs just a little bit less.

I truly believe that without adversity, we cannot reach our ultimate potential. The worst thing we can do for ourselves is to try to avoid, drown, or numb the adversity in our lives. Adversity is the fuel that can catapult us to accomplish things that are beyond our wildest dreams.

Our Deepest Happiness and Self-Fulfillment Can't Be Achieved Without Overcoming Challenges

Aldous Huxley's classic novel *Brave New World* presents a future scenario in which humans are genetically designed to be happy and satisfied in specific life roles. For example, the "alpha" humans are designed for intellectual work and the "epsilons" are designed with a lower intelligence so that they can be satisfied performing mundane yet necessary tasks such as janitorial work.

All of the genetically designed humans live within a walled city of some sort. However, there remain a few "savage reservations" beyond the walls, where the old, imperfect life still continues, complete with struggles and hardships. I read this at the age of seventeen and thought to myself, "Wow, this is great! I'd love to be a part of the genetically modified society. You would never know what you're missing, and you would never have to struggle or suffer mentally, no matter what your caste—whether you were designed for higher or lower intellectual functions."

The book tried to make the point that the "savages" despite their hardships, broken hearts, and daily struggles to make life tolerable were happier than the genetically programmed humans. I didn't buy it. What did I know? I had not yet faced any significant life struggle, and could not possibly understand how powerfully rewarding it feels to overcome a very difficult situation.

Looking back now at age forty-nine, I get it. The deepest sense of self-fulfillment, satisfaction, and happiness comes from taking on a difficult challenge and winning. When you've faced such an overwhelming challenge and asked yourself, "How can I possibly get through this?" and you've dug deep and found a way, how did you feel? If you haven't had the privilege of experiencing this, there are two possible reasons:

1. You've refused to take on challenges and have resigned yourself to live with your current situation; or
2. You haven't yet faced significant challenges. However, I doubt this is the case if you're reading this book.

When those seemingly insurmountable challenges present themselves on your health journey (and I guarantee they will), don't wish them away or try to avoid them. Take them on and risk finding your deepest sense of satisfaction, self-fulfillment, and happiness on the other side.

Applying Resilience to Your Health Champion Journey

If you can fully accept the fact that there is no such thing as being one hundred percent healthy, and that your current health state is not your final destination, that there are always improvements to be made, then you've taken a significant step toward enhancing your ability to persevere. Throughout my journey, there have been so many instances in which I thought "this must be it. I've made so much progress, there can't possibly be anything else out there that can improve my condition." But because I let my WHY lead me, I would continue to explore potential solutions to the pain that crept in as I pushed my body to increasingly higher levels. The words that kept entering my mind were "just maybe." Just maybe there is something more out there that can help me go even further. I would think, "Although there probably isn't much more I can do, I need to keep searching, just in case … " That thought process was directly related to how strongly I wanted to reach my WHY at various stages of my journey.

Your quest to become as healthy as you can be is truly a journey. It will be filled with adventure, adversity, setbacks, and victories. Without a battle, there can be no victory. Get ready to take on the adversity and fight the battles. There are so many physical, emotional, and mental rewards in pushing forward, compared to accepting the current situation.

Ask Yourself "What Is the Lesson in This Setback?"

Just when I thought I had everything figured out with my chronic myofascial pain condition and was training for my first marathon in 2013, I started to develop really bad pain under my feet, which I later discovered was plantar fasciitis. My instinctive response was to tell myself I had reached my limit. This was it. It had been a great ride, but I had taken my flawed body as far as it could go. For a moment, I began to accept that this problem would keep me not only from running the marathon, but also from realizing my dream of completing the IRONMAN triathlon later in the year. However, I quickly shifted my mindset from acceptance to problem-solving. So I began asking myself, "What is the best way to figure this out and deal with it?" I went back to searching and asking questions.

As I pursued the solution to this persistent, painful, and annoying foot problem, it actually led me to uncover further solutions to reduce my overall symptoms associated with chronic myofascial pain syndrome.

My aches and pains and stiffness episodes were creeping in more consistently in the spring and summer of 2013, given all the training for both the marathon (in May) and the IRONMAN (in August). The symptoms would show up in various parts of my body, seeming to work their way up and down or side to side across my body. Although I was getting concerned about the seemingly renewed symptoms of myofascial dysfunction, I had trained myself not to panic at these episodes. After all, at age forty-seven, I was asking more of my body than I ever had in my life. I assumed I was getting close to reaching my absolute physical limit. I just had to focus on all the things I knew could help me: Frequency Specific Microcurrent (FSM)—a therapy based on low-level electrical currents; stretching; strength workouts; self-massage using a roller and ball designed for massaging soft tissues; yoga; Epsom salt baths; ice; chiropractor; and my nutrition plan.

Though it was difficult and painful, I managed to complete the marathon. And through the experience, I figured out that the plantar fasciitis I had been struggling with was related to a right hip problem that surfaced during the marathon. The "side chain" fascia stretches all the way from the neck to under the foot along the entire side of the body. It was the same old problem all over again, just dressed up differently. My running had put more strain than ever on the side chains; the myofascial dysfunction was just manifesting itself as plantar fasciitis this time. At least I knew what I was dealing with, and I continued to look for more answers along the lines of optimizing the functioning of myofascial tissue.

One of the positives that emerged from persevering through the marathon was the thought that improving my running technique could help minimize my foot pain. Running is something we all do from a young age, so we never question whether we're doing it properly. It's one thing to run a few kilometers here and there, but I was pounding out about a hundred kilometers each month at this point. I started to think it might make sense to consult a few experts about my running technique, so I turned to Jillian my exercise physiologist, and to a chiropractor who subspecializes in gait analysis for runners. I learned quite a bit from both of them and began including some running-specific drills into my strength workouts. I also became even more aware of my posture and of using the correct muscles while running.

While attending our triathlon club's fundraising event, I was fortunate enough to sit with Brooke Brown, one of Canada's top female full-distance triathletes. I told her I had signed up for the August 18 Mont-Tremblant IRONMAN event but was a little concerned about my ability to run, given the latest problems with my feet. She recommended getting a floating belt and substituting "water running" for some running workouts; this would allow me to continue using the running muscles without pounding on my feet. So I added this approach to my training, in addition to some recommendations made by a professional bike fitter to minimize strain on the body from cycling. Simply by identifying and implementing additional approaches to managing my problem, my hopes were up again. These, combined with my newly uncovered IV sessions and trigger point injections were giving me the hope I needed to believe I could make it through the IRONMAN—especially the running part.

As a result of continuing to view myself as Chief Problem Solver on a never-ending health-improvement journey, I was able to effectively deal with the foot pain. And as a bonus, I found several more solutions that improved my body's ability to weather the hours of swimming, biking, and running involved in training for and completing an IRONMAN event with minimal myofascial pain symptoms and, most importantly, with no show-stopping injuries.

Looking back, I thought to myself, "It's a good thing that foot problem showed up when it did! It presented me with an opportunity to discover more solutions to my underlying condition in time to be ready for the IRONMAN." The foot pain was a powerful learning opportunity in disguise. As Andre Agassi's trainer and mentor Gil Reyes put it, "There's a whole lot of good on the other side of tired, Andre ... you need to get tired more often." When you feel too tired or sore or frustrated to go on, remember that good things are often hidden on the other side of adversity.

Expectations of Health Champions

I've talked about how important it is to expect that achieving your healthiest potential will be a never-ending journey. Unrealistic expectations like finding a magic bullet can lead to inaction, as can purely negative expectations such as, "It's never going to get any better." To persist on this never-ending and rewarding Health Champion journey means an adjustment of thoughts and behaviors, most of which were covered in Steps 1 through 8. However, within this ninth step focused on never giving up, I'd like to revisit some of the concepts presented in Steps 1 through 8 that tie into key expectations that will contribute to driving you forward on your Health Champion journey.

Give It Time

It takes time for treatments and lifestyle changes to have an impact. If a treatment modality is attempting to get at the root of your health problem, there's a good chance it will take a lot of time before you begin to feel the benefits. You must have a solid grasp of how long you need to implement something before you feel a difference. Good examples are nutritional changes. These can take as long as three or four months before you feel a significant impact. While I attempted some shotgun changes to my diet and added supplements early in the process, I became frustrated and gave up within a few weeks. In addition, I had no professional guidance on what to change and why.

Understanding how and why a behavior change can impact your condition can make a huge difference on your likelihood of persevering with the adjustment.

Work on Weaknesses

If it doesn't feel good it might be what you need. If something recommended by a knowledgeable and trusted health professional isn't comfortable or you feel you "can't" do it, it's probably because you need to do it! You're probably working on a weakness that needs to be strengthened. As long as you're working with someone whom you believe is competent in his or her field, be sure to think twice before making your own judgments about whether certain treatments or exercises are good for you or not. Ask your health professional for a rationale as to why you should continue doing something that doesn't feel good to you. Getting a satisfactory answer to this question could save you years of pain and distress if it compels you to implement something that ultimately works.

Tackle Adversity

It's going to be hard. There is no magic bullet. Expect and accept that you have a significant challenge ahead of you. Not only do you have to locate the pieces of your health puzzle, you have to figure out how they fit together. In addition, you have to muster up the strength and courage to tackle adversity. As I sat with a group of seven highly intelligent, motivated, and fit women recently, some of them shared stories of how they overcame difficult situations to arrive at very rewarding outcomes. Hearing these reinforced for me the power of the message found in *The Adversity Advantage* by Paul Stoltz.

The women in the group shared the achievements that they were most proud of—these included getting out of bad relationships and regaining control of their lives after battling and overcoming negative health experiences. We all agreed that we were stronger and better for having overcome a difficult situation. It would have been easier at the time to just keep the status quo rather than muster up the courage to take on the challenge. But without the fight, we never would have been able to experience the same level of self-fulfillment.

The bottom line is that by taking on a very difficult situation, and "pushing through" the adversity rather than shying away from it and letting it take over, we can arrive at a better place than if we had never faced the adversity. My experience has proven that to me. Had I not battled and overcome chronic myofascial pain syndrome, I almost certainly would have gone through life believing that completing an IRONMAN was completely out of reach for me. What's more, I might have remained in the corporate job I hated rather than taking on the challenge of writing my first book and starting a business based on my passion and purpose.

When adversity strikes, ask yourself these two questions to get activated:

- WHY is it important to me to take on this adversity and get to a better place? This is a critical question to ask yourself. Fighting adversity is hard. You need an emotionally compelling reason to do it. Is it to regain your dignity? Is it to honor a loved one? Is it to teach your kids about not giving up?
- What is the pain of NOT doing anything about it, and letting the adversity take over? Really feel that pain. It might be enough to drive you into action. But remember that this negative push is only the ignition. The WHY is the force that keeps you moving forward, even when you've run out of gas.

It's a Never-Ending Journey

It's a process, an iterative loop. There is no final destination, so you might as well enjoy the journey.

Just as you will need to do, I have to keep reminding myself that this journey of mine never ends. It's an ongoing pilgrimage of discovery, and that's what makes it so exhilarating. Once you stop the search, you deprive yourself of the possibility of reaching new levels of wellness. On several occasions, I believed I had reached my limit. However, using adversity as fuel to uncover more solutions, I was able to keep pushing far beyond what I believed was possible for my body.

I recently revisited the importance of strictly adhering to the nutrition plan that was designed for me in 2010. I know that the nutrition plan was a big part of the dramatic improvement in my symptoms. But over time, I had let myself drift a little from the strict guidelines, allowing myself to eat processed carbohydrates that include gluten. Perhaps not so coincidentally, some of my symptoms crept back over an eighteen-month period. When I started to research the possible association of gluten with myofascial symptoms, I found some interesting information. There is evidence that gluten and other food intolerances can be linked to "muscle stiffness" and various myofascial pain disorders.

On my dad's side of the family, there were several members with myofascial symptoms (stiffness, cramping, etc.), and one of his cousins had celiac disease (extreme gluten intolerance). This got me thinking seriously about the real possibility that one of the underlying drivers of my symptoms is gluten intolerance. Celiac disease is an autoimmune disorder that results in damage to the small intestine. I've recently learned that a large proportion of people with the condition have a "silent" form of it, and have no serious gastrointestinal symptoms.[22] However, there are many other symptoms associated with celiac disease, including iron deficiency and musculoskeletal symptoms—both of which I suffer from.

The only effective treatment for celiac disease is a strictly gluten-free diet. It can take several months of strict adherence to a gluten-free diet for symptoms to improve and for the small intestine to heal. Although I never pursued a diagnosis of celiac disease, I have a family history and the knowledge that the only cure is a gluten-free diet. So I decided to take the gluten-free challenge by completely removing gluten from my diet and have been adhering to my nutrition plan for the past seven months. I've felt a gradual and significant reduction in the overall levels of chronic muscle stiffness, and I am planning to have my iron levels retested in the near future. I am also considering a full blood screening for all food intolerances for myself and for my family. You can find various companies out there providing these types of screenings, often in conjunction with naturopathic, pharmacy, or other health services. Some diagnostic providers offer convenient online access to comprehensive health screenings including heart disease, cancer, diabetes, inflammation, hormone imbalance, thyroid irregularity, and food intolerance tests for over two hundred of the most common food sensitivities.

Although these food sensitivity screening tests are imperfect, I believe that some information is better than operating in the dark. You might also want to think about exploring the possible nutritional links to your condition. If nothing else, you will become more informed about the impact of your nutritional choices on your overall health and vitality.

Keep learning and implementing. Enjoy the process.

---

[22] Articles about celiac disease: todaysdietitian.com/newarchives/050114p22.shtml; and Green P.H. "The many faces of celiac disease: clinical presentation of celiac disease in the adult population." *Gastroenterology.* 2005;128:S74–S78

The Importance of Continuing the Search: An Illustration

The news reporter declared it a "miracle." A sixty-eight-year-old man who was severely visually impaired almost his whole life (since the 1940s), met a doctor who offered him cataract surgery at a Montreal hospital after he was hospitalized there for a fall. After the cataracts were removed, he was miraculously able to see clearly for the first time in his life. But people in Canada have undergone successful cataract surgeries since the 1970s! Why was this man living in blindness these last forty years since effective surgery had been developed?

Although I do not have any details on this man's history, my best guess is that he gave up hope of finding a solution after several unsuccessful surgeries in his youth (up until the 1960s). And if he saw a family doctor in the last four decades, it's obvious that the doctor was not offering any solutions without the patient asking questions.

With the existence of a common and successful treatment for his problem, this man should have been able to see the world around him for at least the past thirty years. Instead he lived in darkness and his life was much more difficult than it needed to be.[23]

So don't give up on researching your condition and continuing to ask questions of as many healthcare professionals as you can find who might be more knowledgeable than average about your particular condition. Tests, treatments, and knowledge-sharing among professionals continue to evolve. If you don't keep asking questions and seeking people with potential solutions, you might miss out on years of improved life quality. No one is going to offer you solutions on a silver platter. You must take charge and seek the answers.

---

[23]The full story can be found on the CBC news website: cbc.ca/news/canada/montreal/montreal-man-68-gets-to-see-for-the-first-time-1.1404097

In Chapter 7, I talked about the importance of understanding and implementing solutions offered by credible, knowledgeable, and problem-solving health professionals. This is one of the keys to perseverance. However, the opposite is also true. When you follow directions precisely and for the recommended time period with no sign of improvement, you must take action. Not only do you need to provide the feedback to the health professional who made the recommendation, but you need to probe into why the intervention(s) is not helping. The more you understand, the better you can explain the situation to other health professionals who can bring a different perspective to solving the problem.

SECTION III—SUMMARY

Whether you think of yourself as someone who has a strong tendency to persevere or not, if you can confidently check the boxes associated with each of the steps below, you're well on your way to making perseverance a natural part of your health-improvement process. And as such, you are increasing the odds of fulfilling your potential.

Step 7: Fully Implement Potential Solutions

- ☐ When a trusted health professional suggests certain approaches to address my health issue, I will inquire about how and why that particular approach could help me.
- ☐ I will ask how long I need to continue a treatment or exercise before I can assess its effectiveness.
- ☐ When presented with new recommendations, I will consider adding them to my current regime of treatments rather than replacing anything, unless I am counselled otherwise.

Step 8: Find Everyday Motivators to Keep You Going

- ☐ I've identified the things that can draw strong, positive emotions by helping me make the connection with my WHY.
- ☐ I've taken action by building a playlist and/or selecting and displaying images that can spur me into action.

Step 9: Never, Ever Give Up

- ☐ I recognize and accept that there is no such destination as one hundred percent health.
- ☐ I welcome adversity as the fuel that can propel me to reach greater heights than I ever dreamed of.
- ☐ Since "healthy" is a never-ending learning journey, I will continuously be on the lookout for approaches that can drive me even further along toward fulfilling my potential.

SECTION IV

On Chronic Pain and Triathlons

The goal of this section is to provide you with some specific information on my experience with chronic myofascial pain syndrome—what it is and what key interventions allowed me to conquer it. I also want to share how participating in triathlons was a fantastic way of motivating me to take action for improving my condition, all the way through to the emotional experience of crossing the finish line at an IRONMAN event. I provide a number of tips on getting started in triathlon, just in case you've caught the bug after reading this book.

Ten

How I Overcame Chronic Myofascial Pain Syndrome

Never give up, for that is just the place and time that the tide will turn.
Harriet Beecher Stowe

If you suffer from chronic pain, generally defined as pain lasting more than three months, you're not alone. A large, nationally representative survey by the American Pain Society found that approximately 30 percent of the US adult population suffers from some form of chronic pain.[24] Two sources of Canadian data found that 20 percent to 30 percent of the Canadian adult population suffers from chronic pain.[25] In all studies, pain was reported at a higher rate among women and with increasing age. I think it's safe to say that no matter what the source of chronic pain is, the problem has not been addressed in a satisfactory way at all within our North American healthcare systems.

Describing Chronic Myofascial Pain Syndrome

Most people with chronic myofascial pain have actually never heard of that condition. I've lived with it for eighteen years and saw the term for the first time about three years ago. There is also a lot of talk about fibromyalgia in the medical literature, which appears to have very similar symptoms. Regardless of

---

[24] ncbi.nlm.nih.gov/pubmed/20797916

[25] ncbi.nlm.nih.gov/pmc/articles/PMC3298051; and statcan.gc.ca/pub/82-003-x/2008001/article/10514-eng.htm

the label, those of us with the condition would describe our symptoms as "chronically stiff and sore muscles, combined with chronic fatigue." The fatigue is likely caused by the stress of suffering through the day and the disturbed sleep caused by pain and discomfort. In my case, not only were my muscles stiff and sore all the time, but I was always on the verge of a new injury as I tried to remain as physically active as possible. Stiffness led to soft tissue injuries, which led to inflammation, which led to more chronic pain in the form of trigger points (muscle "knots"). The result was pain, discomfort, misery, and depression.

One of the reasons this condition is not better recognized or understood by the medical community is because there is no recognized medical specialty that "owns" muscles and connective tissues. I saw a few dozen physicians about my condition over the course of thirteen years, and the only relief I got was from a physiotherapist and a massage therapist who understood the concept of myofascial trigger points. But these were very short-lived bouts of relief that did not address the underlying issues. Why were my soft tissues as hard as rock and tied up in knots in the first place? No amount of massage or trigger point release could be sustained until we figured out what was behind the tissue dysfunction.

A trigger point is an area within the muscle where overstimulated muscle contraction cells (sarcomeres) become unable to release their contracted state. This contracted state results in restricted blood flow to the area of the muscle. This sends a pain signal to the brain, which in turn signals the muscle to stop working. This unused muscle then begins to shorten and tighten up, which leads to the feeling of stiffness and "pulling." When this reaches the chronic stage (sustained over time), not only do the muscles feel stiff and tight all the time, but weaknesses develop in various areas across the body. This leads to imbalances, which then put the sufferer at risk for soft tissue injuries with each sudden or strenuous movement. These injuries can lead to more trigger points, and the cycle of misery goes on. The cycle of misery lasted thirteen years for me. Although I've had several breakthroughs and major improvements over the last five years, I continue to learn about additional ways to reduce symptoms and improve my quality of life.

One of the most frustrating things about chronic myofascial pain syndrome is that even if a healthcare practitioner finds a way of releasing a specific trigger point in one muscle, this could lead to stressing other muscles in a related muscle group. In other words, there can be a sort of chain reaction among muscles up and down and across the body, so that you never seem to get to the cause of the problem. There have been so many times when I have been sure of the origin of the problem, had the trigger points released in that area by my chiropractor, then woken up the next day with pain in the corresponding muscles on the other side of my body! However, with patience and some good people on your team who are experienced in treating and addressing the various aspects of myofascial issues, you can make some remarkable progress.

Approaches That Led to Improvements in My Condition

Below are some of the key lifestyle modifications and treatments that led me from chronic pain, frustration, and debilitation to hope and new levels of physical achievement. These approaches worked for me; however, please involve knowledgeable problem-solving health professionals in the process of identifying and trying various approaches that could work for you.

Nutrition

As it turns out, the key to addressing the underlying soft tissue dysfunction was a nutritional and supplement plan designed to optimize soft tissue function. This step is the foundation required to allow the other treatments and approaches to have a lasting effect on myofascial tissues. Depletion of minerals such as magnesium can be associated with soft tissue disorders like fibromyalgia and chronic myofascial pain. And it can take a long time to not only repair the underlying problems that are contributing to the low levels of minerals in the body, but also to replenish the missing minerals.

In my research on this issue, I've uncovered some interesting insights about why and how modern day humans have become depleted of minerals.[26] I share some of these with you below as food for thought. Mineral deficiency is quite common all over the world, in part, because of modern-day living. Our soil has been depleted of minerals, resulting in fewer mineral-rich types of produce on supermarket shelves.

Some Causes of Mineral Depletion in Humans

Soil Depletion

This is the number one reason that most people are mineral deficient. Soil depletion over time has been well documented by the US government (see the graph in the first article in footnote 26). Even organically grown vegetables are lacking in minerals—organic farming most typically only addresses the pesticide/chemical issues. The best way to get mineral-rich fruits and vegetables is through bio-dynamic produce, local CSAs (Community Supported Agriculture groups) that practice crop rotation and soil supplementation through compost and other means, and of course growing your own

---

[26]Three useful links are a) http://preventdisease.com/news/12/090712_18-Causes-of-Mineral-Depletion.shtml

b) scientificamerican.com/article/soil-depletion-and-nutrition-loss; and

c) divinehealthfromtheinsideout.com/2012/05/factors-that-deplete-minerals-from-the-body

garden, which allows you to work on the integrity of the soil.[27] Not to mention, the animals we consume need to be raised on good quality pastures with good soil conditions as well.

Alcohol

The excretion of magnesium through the kidneys is accelerated with alcohol consumption. It can also deplete calcium, zinc, iron, manganese, potassium, and chromium.

Antacids and Acid Blockers

These deplete calcium, but people are often unaware because testing is done on blood levels, and only 1 percent of the calcium in the body is in the blood. This doesn't indicate the loss in the bones/tissues. Antacids and acid blockers reduce stomach acid levels, which reduces the body's ability to break down and absorb minerals, specifically calcium.

Birth Control Pills

These deplete magnesium and zinc, along with numerous other vitamins. And since they have a direct impact on our hormones this also plays with our ability to get the minerals needed. They can be associated with zinc depletion by causing an excess retention of copper in the body, which competes with the absorption of zinc.

Coffee and Other Caffeine-Containing Drinks

Calcium and magnesium are lost in our urine with the diuretic effect of coffee. Potassium and sodium will be lost as well.

---

[27]Community Supported Agriculture programs are particular networks or associations of individuals who have pledged to support one or more local farms, with growers and consumers sharing the risks and benefits of food production.

Corticosteroids Such as Cortisone

These prescription drugs are used to control pain and inflammation, and with prolonged use can contribute to severe calcium loss. They also deplete potassium. Many other prescription pharmaceuticals are involved in depleting the body of various nutrients.

Excess Grains

Phytic acid found in most grains binds with the minerals in the intestine and blocks absorption, causing the minerals to be excreted unused.

Heavy Metal Toxicity

The mercury found in amalgam fillings and in certain fish blocks magnesium and zinc absorption. Mercury binds with magnesium and renders it inaccessible to the body. Aluminum found in antacids, antiperspirants, cosmetics, and aluminum foil penetrates the blood-brain barrier and is very difficult to detoxify. It also impedes the utilization of calcium, magnesium, and phosphorous.

Hyperthyroidism

This condition causes increased calcium losses and increased calcium resorption (withdrawal) from the bone. This creates the need for more magnesium, thus resulting in magnesium depletion as well.

Radiation

Any type of electromagnetic frequency has an effect on the body's ability to absorb and assimilate minerals.

Soft Drinks

These contain excess phosphorous, which leads to reduced body storage of calcium because phosphorous and calcium compete for absorption in the intestines. Soda also causes potassium loss.

The Standard American Diet (S.A.D.)

The excess phosphorous found in this typical diet low in fresh foods and high in refined and processed foods causes depletion of calcium, which has been shown to cause bone loss. Magnesium, chromium, and many other minerals are also lost in processing.

Sugar

Magnesium is wasted in processing high sugar foods. I've read that for every molecule of sugar consumed, our bodies use anywhere from 28 to 54 molecules of magnesium to process it. Sugar also depletes potassium and chromium.

Although minerals themselves play a critical role in our bodies, we can't ignore the specific cofactors that help them work properly. These cofactors are found alongside minerals in whole foods, thus ensuring the minerals are used effectively by the body.

The best way to ensure you are getting a wide array of minerals is by eating a nutrient-dense diet of properly prepared whole foods.

After several months on my customized nutrition plan, the massages, exercises, and chiropractic treatments seemed to have a much more pronounced and lasting effect. Find a clinical or holistic nutritionist who specializes in sports nutrition and/or musculoskeletal conditions. He or she should guide you on general principles to follow in order to optimize soft tissue function and should also recommend blood work that can be used to tailor a nutrition plan to your specific needs. For me, the general principles included much more protein than I was eating, about a hundred percent more fish, the elimination of sugar and processed carbohydrates, and a dramatic increase in all things green and crunchy. A key underlying principle is to avoid foods that cause insulin spikes. It's hard to go wrong if I stay away from sugars and processed grains, and I maximize whole foods such as organic meats, fruits, vegetables, and legumes. Following is a partial list of what's "in" and what's "out" of my nutrition plan.

What's IN:

- all vegetables, especially dark green leafy ones
- most fruit, with berries and citrus fruit being at the top of the list
- fish—mainly wild pacific salmon, haddock, canned light tuna, and other fish with low levels of mercury—2 to 3 ounces almost every day[28]
- lean organic meats—mainly chicken and turkey—with a maximum of 2 to 3 small servings of red meat per week
- yogurt with protein powder
- beans
- nuts (I can't eat these due to allergies, but good choices if you're not allergic)
- chia, hemp heart, pumpkin, and sunflower seeds

What's OUT:

- most breads (the only one I've discovered that is acceptable is chia bread)

---

[28]For details on types of fish and corresponding mercury levels, refer to fda.gov/food/foodborneillnesscontaminants/metals/ucm115644.htm; and hc-sc.gc.ca/fn-an/securit/chem-chim/environ/mercur/cons-adv-etud-eng.php

- most pasta (although I found a good one with high protein made of 100 percent legumes at tolerantfoods.com)
- any and all processed sugar and sweets
- fruit juices
- cakes, cookies, crackers, and so on

Given my recent discoveries about the likely link between gluten and my myofascial dysfunction (as described in Chapter 9), when I do feel like treating myself and breaking a few nutrition rules, I just make sure that I choose gluten-free options.

Beyond Nutrition—Additional Approaches

Magnesium

As discussed previously, magnesium plays an important role in soft tissue function. You should know your magnesium level. If it is anywhere near the bottom of the reference range, I encourage you to take a daily magnesium supplement. You should also be aware that blood levels of magnesium are not that accurate in determining whether your tissues are getting enough of the mineral. Consult with a knowledgeable health professional to determine whether your symptoms could be improved with a magnesium supplement, and what the right dose is for you.

Omega-3 Supplements

The evidence on omega-3 fatty acids is mounting in terms of their role in protecting against heart disease, eye disease, and inflammatory conditions. It is important to ingest these by eating certain fish, nuts, and good quality oils. However, because I want to gain the maximum anti-inflammatory effect provided by omega-3 fatty acids, in addition to eating five to seven fish servings per week (one serving being 2 or 3 ounces),

I take a supplement that is high in pure EPA and DHA, the two omega-3 fatty acids associated with the greatest benefits.

Antioxidants

Although many products claim to contain antioxidants, the ultimate aim is to increase the amount of glutathione, the master antioxidant produced by our bodies. Maximizing the glutathione in your system is critical to having a healthy immune system that can fight off whatever life throws at it. No matter what product you choose as an antioxidant aid and immune booster, verify that it has been clinically proven to increase glutathione levels in humans. The product I've found to have the best data behind it is Immunocal® by Immunotec. You can check it out at immunotec.com. I take one or two packets a day mixed with plain or vanilla yogurt.

Iron

I've been taking an iron supplement since 2011, when I discovered my iron stores were almost completely depleted. Although I'm not certain whether low iron is related to my myofascial pain symptoms, I'm convinced it is linked to the underlying condition that was causing all the pain and stiffness. If the problem is related to poor absorption of minerals like magnesium from the intestines, then it makes sense that iron would be poorly absorbed as well. As you know, iron is critical in transporting oxygen to your cells. Low iron will contribute to low energy and fatigue. If you feel you don't have sufficient energy to get through the day, let alone take on an exercise program, ask your doctor, nurse practitioner, or other health professional to check your iron levels.

Keep in mind that I never got a call from my doctor's office the first time my iron was checked in 2010. It was when I approached my doctor specifically about almost passing out at a triathlon that he pulled the file and noticed how low the iron level was. Remember that if your number falls somewhere within the "reference range" and the lab doesn't flag your result as being in the low range, you won't get a call from your doctor. So be proactive and ask for a review of your results no matter what. And it doesn't end there. After three or four months of taking an oral supplement of iron, have your iron levels checked again. Mine hardly went up after taking very high doses in pill form for four months. I had to get iron injections in order to see a significant rise. This reinforces my hunch about the fact that my gut was not properly absorbing the iron.

Hydration

It took a while for me to understand the true concept of hydration. Unless sufficient water is accessing your tissues on an ongoing basis, you are not hydrated. Drinking water when you're thirsty does not mean you're hydrated. Everyone's body deals with water and electrolytes differently. Key electrolytes for optimal soft tissue function are calcium, magnesium, potassium, and sodium. If your intestines are inflamed or not doing their job properly for whatever reason, there's a risk that these electrolytes aren't being fully absorbed from your diet. This highlights the importance of a nutrition and supplement plan tailored to your body's specific needs. It also reinforces the fact that a diet high in processed foods and sugar, which depletes us of minerals (many of which are key electrolytes), should simply be avoided by anyone who wants to optimize their health.

I've learned over many years that my body requires not only three liters of water per day, but I also need to take an electrolyte drink each day. And when I'm working out hard and sweating, I need to add one liter of a combination of water and electrolyte drink per hour of workout. I recommend talking to a knowledgeable pharmacist (ideally affiliated with a sports medicine clinic) about high quality electrolyte drinks. The ones most advertised might not necessarily be the best. In addition, I discovered intravenous (IV) electrolytes, which can flood the body with electrolytes that are being depleted faster than they can be replenished with drinks alone. This is especially important during periods of heavy training. I've figured out that part of the reason for my chronic myofascial condition is that my body seems to be naturally low in electrolytes, meaning the tissues can be chronically dehydrated. Endurance training depletes my body of these precious electrolytes, and sometimes the volume of electrolyte drink required for replenishment is too much for my stomach to take, so the IV does the trick. The clinic I go to is called Vitamindrip®, and the IVs are directed by a trained naturopath. As a bonus, the IV can also be loaded with amino acids, antioxidants, and other nutrients that are beneficial to your soft tissues. After these IV treatments, I can feel the stiffness melting away.

Strength Training Program

As mentioned previously, it was an exercise physiologist who truly turned things around for me. It was her holistic approach (recommending looking at blood biochemistry, nutrition, supplements, and chiropractic care) in addition to developing a strength and flexibility program that took me from dysfunctional to functional. The customized strength and flexibility training program was a pivotal component of my recovery plan, as was Jillian's clear explanations of *why* I had to do all the exercises she included in my program. It was the first time someone made me realize that uncomfortable exercises were critical to "wake up" weak muscles and stiff tissues in order to get me to the next level. Remember, no strength program should ever feel comfortable. If it does, then you are not getting stronger!

Don't take the easy route and just hire any trainer at your

nearby gym. Look for someone with the Certified Exercise Physiologist (CEP) designation from the Canadian Society for Exercise Physiologists or the Certified Strength and Conditioning Specialist (CSCS) designation from the National Strength and Conditioning Association (US). There might be other designations and/or knowledgeable trainers and strength coaches out there, but it is difficult to sort out the true experts without the higher-level certifications. Generally speaking, you want to make sure that as a minimum they have a degree in a science like kinesiology, in addition to specialized training for strength coaching. Ideally, they are affiliated with sports medicine clinics and/or sports organizations. Remember, you do not have to be an athlete to hire these people; you just have to want to work with someone knowledgeable enough to have been selected by a sports medicine clinic or a sports team.

Yoga

Every time I walk out of a yoga class, I feel relaxed, taller, and younger! I highly recommend giving yoga a solid try. This means at least one class per week for a few months. Notice how you feel after each class. I recommend starting with the slower flowing classes such as hatha, yin, or basic vinyasa. If you tend to be very stiff or inflexible, I recommend a studio that conducts its classes in a hot or warm room. Do your homework on the yoga studio. Be wary of "yoga" classes at the neighborhood gym or community center. Ask for the types of credentials the facility requires when hiring yoga instructors. One important clue that indicates a high quality studio is the fact that they regularly conduct teacher training. You can also inquire about which of their instructors teach other yoga instructors, and whether all their instructors take part in ongoing training.

Chiropractic Care/Acupuncture

A chiropractor's office (especially one affiliated with a sports medicine clinic) is a great place to start with any musculoskeletal problem. Many chiropractors also practice acupuncture, which is one of the treatments that my chiropractor uses on me. Active Release Therapy (ART) has also proven very effective for me and is practiced by many chiropractors. I get a lot of relief from both stiffness and pain after a chiropractic session involving both acupuncture and ART.

Frequency Specific Microcurrent (FSM)

FSM is a treatment modality based on low levels of electrical current programmed to match the type of tissue and the type of disorder being addressed. It has helped me immensely, and I still use it several times per week. If you're interested in the details of applying the therapy, you can read the book, *Frequency Specific Microcurrent in Pain Management* developed by Doctor of Chiropractic, Dr. Carolyn McMakin.[29] Dr. McMakin has studied the effects of FSM treatment on multiple health conditions in thousands of patients. My takeaway from her book is that myofascial pain is one of the most responsive to FSM therapy. In fact, she says if there is no improvement in pain with the FSM myofascial treatment protocols, then there is a good possibility that the pain is not myofascial.[30] The two practitioners I've met who are most knowledgeable about FSM are an osteopath and a chiropractor. Since FSM is not a mainstream treatment, you will likely need to do your research on practitioners who are familiar with it and have the equipment. I found it so helpful when used regularly (several protocols per week) that I invested in my own portable machine, which I use under the direction of an osteopath.

---

[29]Elsevier Ltd, 2011

[30]You can also find a more layman-friendly write-up on FSM to discuss with your health professionals at naturopathic-physician.com/index.php?page=41.

Massage

Whether it is with a highly credentialed massage therapist or on your own with a roller or massage ball, massage can make a big difference in your life, especially if you're doing the hydration, nutrition, and supplements right. The nutrition and hydration set the stage that will allow your soft tissues to benefit the most from massage therapy. About 95 percent of my massage therapy is self-administered with a ball and roller. It's great to see my fantastic massage therapist, Tonya, on occasion, but given my busy schedule it is more realistic for me to do my own massaging at home. I tend to spend about fifteen minutes on it before going to bed. It allows me to get to sleep faster by taking care of the nagging tight spots that pop up during the day.

Osteopathy

Although I only recently discovered the benefits of the discipline of osteopathy, I realize that a good osteopath can also help me a great deal with musculoskeletal complaints by further addressing the pain and stiffness. If you can find an osteopathic practitioner with other credentials (for example, Registered Massage Therapist, Structural Integrationist) to their name, it's a pretty good bet that they are deep into understanding and solving soft tissue problems. My osteopath is one of those gifted practitioners who deeply understands myofascial issues.

Trigger Point Injections

This is another treatment that could be worth exploring. If you always feel like your muscles are tight and "lumpy," you might have trigger points that could be released with an injection of vitamin B12 or another innocuous solution selected by the administering practitioner. I can feel the tight trigger points releasing almost immediately after receiving the injections, and the improvement can last for weeks or more. This would be something worth asking a sports medicine physician or another health professional specializing in musculoskeletal conditions about. General practitioners may or may not be familiar with trigger point injections.

Good Quality Sleep

If you have been told you snore a lot and/or wake up frequently during the night, I recommend you ask your doctor about being tested for sleep apnea. As mentioned in Chapter 5, sleep apnea is a condition in which the throat closes causing reduced oxygen supply to the body, and is associated with a negative impact on soft tissues, the heart, and the brain. You should be referred for a consultation with a sleep specialist in order to be properly tested for apnea. If you do have apnea, you'll likely be told, as I was, that the most effective treatment is a CPAP machine (described in Chapter 5). If you can manage to use the CPAP every night, then it's clearly the best choice. However, if you're like me and you can't handle having a tube connected to your face, you should look into a custom dental appliance designed to keep the jaw in a position that limits the likelihood of the throat closing.

Epsom Salt Baths

Whether it's the Epsom salts or the hot water (or a combination), I usually feel pretty good the morning after having soaked for fifteen to twenty minutes the night before in a nice hot bath with two cups of Epsom salts dissolved in it. I couldn't find any high quality scientific evidence that Epsom salts can relax muscles or relieve muscle pain, but they certainly can't hurt. The only caveat is that I need to drink a lot of water before, during, and/or after an Epsom salt bath, since I find that the salt water tends to dehydrate me. While you might not have lots of spare time to soak in a hot bath, consider using it as reading time. I've never soaked in the tub without a book in hand; it would feel much too unproductive!

Heat

In addition to hot baths, I often go to bed with a heating pad on the part of my body that feels tight that day. It makes a difference for me and I encourage you to give it a try if your main complaint is stiffness.

Ice

In my experience, the type of musculoskeletal pain caused by myofascial pain syndrome can usually be reduced with icing. I can often be seen walking around the house with an ice pack strapped to a body part that feels uncomfortable or irritated, and it usually provides relief. Look for reusable freezer packs and Velcro-equipped cloth holders that you can strap on to the painful body part. I generally leave the ice on for ten minutes at a time. The nice thing about the reusable ice packs is that they warm up over time, making it unlikely that you will overdo the cold.

Find What Works for You

This long list of interventions might seem a bit overwhelming to you, but I'm just putting all the options out there so you can start looking into what might work for you. Chances are two to four of the above approaches could be critical for you and your particular situation. You just need to start with identifying at least one and building on it. Several of these approaches will require some financial investment, but you'd be surprised how you can find the funding when you identify something that liberates you from pain and discomfort.

Start taking action today. There are many questions to be asked, and lots of information to gather that probably won't be offered up by your family doctor. Your best chance is to start with a clinic that specializes in sports medicine and integrates various health professionals like chiropractors, massage therapists, physiotherapists, nutritionists, exercise physiologists, and other professionals trained to optimize musculoskeletal functioning.

Eleven

Triathlon—The Perfect Vehicle for My Health Recovery Journey

You miss one hundred percent of the shots you don't take.
Wayne Gretzky

If you think perfect health is required to participate in triathlons or any other sport for which you have a passion, think again! Committing to the right sport can motivate you to search for solutions to your health challenges. Then step-by-step, you might find yourself accomplishing things beyond your wildest dreams.

I loved tennis and running, but during my thirteen-year chronic pain struggle, frequent injuries prevented me from doing much of these high impact sports. My fragile body, riddled with stiffness, muscle "knots," chronic pain, and frequent soft tissue injuries like muscle tears and tendinitis couldn't handle the pounding anymore. I was beginning to give up on being as active as I wanted to be.

Staying Active Despite Having a Fragile Body

As I began working on solving my chronic pain issues and rehabilitating my body through nutritional changes, strength training, yoga, chiropractic, and other approaches, my friend suggested I join her in a swimming class. I hesitantly agreed, convincing myself it was a low impact sport that could be sustainable despite my history of chronic injuries. The only problem was that I was a terrible swimmer! After one lap of the 25 meter pool at the first swim class, I was totally out of breath. I felt completely out of my league. But I had found a new challenge. There was nowhere to go but up with this swimming thing!

I persevered with the swimming, joining a swim club that included several triathletes in the membership. This made me think, "Maybe bike riding would be okay on my body." So I began riding the stationary bike at the gym and bought a hybrid bike with the thought of maybe entering a Sprint Distance triathlon event in the near future. The only issue was that triathlons involve running, and running caused me injuries. However, as my health improved with the implementation of my strength program, nutrition plan, and treatments from a sports chiropractor, I began to believe that one day my body might be able to handle running some short distances. So I signed up for my first sprint triathlon at the age of forty-three, after thirteen years of struggling with chronic myofascial pain syndrome.

Getting to My First Triathlon

My race training generally involved swimming (until I pulled a shoulder muscle two months before the race), cycling (the only thing I could do regularly up until race day), and the elliptical trainer (as I had also pulled a calf muscle during a training run six weeks prior to the race, I couldn't run). I seriously wondered if I should be showing up at all to this race. Since I had nothing to lose, and it might be the only one I ever signed up for, I decided to go for it. It was one of the scariest days of my life. Not only was I an undertrained, marginal swimmer, this was to be my first open-water swim! I kept telling myself "If you can make it out of the water within the cut-off time, you can finish this thing." I could always walk the run course if necessary.

I was incredibly nervous driving myself to the race (Rod and the kids were about ninety minutes behind me). But there is an indescribable power in believing this could be your only chance to do something physically challenging that you never thought you could even come close to. In my mind, this was *it*. If I could just finish this race, I would be satisfied, knowing I had pushed myself to the limit. In fact, I had three very clear goals for this race:

1.   Don't develop any new injuries or worsen existing injuries.
2.   Finish the race.
3.   Don't be last in my age group (which at that point wouldn't have mattered as long as #1 and #2 were achieved).

Walking from the parking lot to the race site was intimidating, with lots of people looking like "real" triathletes. There I was with my $700 hybrid bike surrounded by expensive racing bikes. I had carefully read all the pre-race instructions, so I got my bike on the rack in the right place and went to the various stations to receive my race number, swim cap, and body markings.

This was my first time putting on a wetsuit. I had rented one from a triathlon shop in Toronto after deciding at the last minute that it might be a good idea. As it turned out, the wetsuit was one of the key factors that allowed me to get through the swim. Lake Ontario was 70° Fahrenheit. For perspective, I don't swim in my pool if it's less than 87° F! I put on the wetsuit backwards and then realized the zipper goes in the back.

As the start time approached, I placed myself in the rear outside corner of the swim pack. The huge body of water that is Lake Ontario scared me to death; it looked really dark and the waves were significant, thanks to the unsettled weather. The buoys were arranged in such a way that I would have to round three corners before heading back into shore. The first buoy looked impossibly far away. My heart rate was over 120 beats per minute before even starting the swim.

Waiting for the start, I spotted Rod and the kids on shore, as well as my brother Mike and his wife, Kerry. Boy, was I glad to see them. The start gun went off, and I started to swim front crawl. This lasted about 50 m (about two minutes), then I had to turn on my back. I started to panic and told myself that there was no way I could get through this swim. I did a few strokes of the elementary backstroke ("frog kick"). I was ready to put my hand up to be rescued by a lifeguard, which would have ended my race. Knowing that Rod and the kids were watching, however, made me think I should give it a harder try. So I went back to doing the front crawl for about 25 m or less at a time, alternating onto my back every 25 m to 50 m.

Before I knew it, I was pretty close to making the turn at the first buoy, and the next stretch to the second buoy was quite a bit shorter than the distance I had just completed. "Okay, so maybe I can make it to the second turn," I thought. Continuing with mainly breaststroke and elementary backstroke, I somehow made it to the second turn. By this point, I thought again about raising my hand to be rescued, and I could see one of the lifeguards looking at me with concern. Once again, I thought about Rod and the kids, my brother and his wife. "If I can just get through this part, then I know I can do the bike and the run (or walk)." Looking ahead, it was one more long stretch followed by a slight turn at the last buoy, and I could see my way to the shore! "Okay, I have to do this. I don't care if it's elementary backstroke all the way." People from the next start group were passing me. When I finally made it out of the water, I felt dizzy and disoriented, but ecstatic! "I did it! I got out!"

When I got to the transition area, I tried to remove my wetsuit. I don't know if it was shock, exhaustion, or cold (probably a combination), but my arms and hands had no strength at all, and I could not even begin to pull off the wetsuit! So I waited a few minutes and tried again. I kept working at it until my strength came back, and I was finally able to pull it off. Then I felt a sense of total freedom. "I did it! I made it in before the swim cut-off time, pulled the wetsuit off, and now I know I can finish this race."

For the first half of the 25 km bike ride, I was so happy that I really didn't pay attention to the fact that it was a race and not a little jaunt through the park. I sort of woke up with about 10 km left and tried to go a little faster. After the bike, I took a few minutes in transition to stretch and improve my chances of running rather than walking the 7 km. To my surprise, I ended up running almost all of it. When I hit the 6 km mark, I thought to myself, "This is never going to end, so just accept the suffering and shut your brain off." I entered a sort of cruise control, which can also be called "the zone." I wasn't even looking for the finish line when I rounded a corner and there it was! There were my husband, kids, brother, and sister-in-law all cheering for me!

It's very difficult to explain the emotions as I crossed that finish line. Exhilaration comes to mind. Gratitude, relief, and pride also come to mind. I started crying, gasped for air, and hugged my support crew. Two hours and twenty-four minutes. Monumental!

When it was all over, my five-year-old daughter asked me, "Did you win, Mommy?"

I paused for a second and answered, "Yes, sweetie. I won *my* race."

This was truly the greatest victory of my life to this point. It was my breakthrough moment. One of the most powerful drivers that made me show up that morning was the thought that, given that my body was beginning to fail again, this could realistically be my only opportunity to participate in a triathlon.

I now truly understood the meaning of having a "stretch goal," something you're not really sure you can accomplish, but you surrender to that little glimmer of hope in your mind and to the voice that says, "Just maybe I can." What if we looked at all stretch goals that way? Life is so unpredictable that any undertaking could be our last for whatever reason.

What transpired on that day was one of the most powerful experiences of my life. Not only did I complete the swim despite considering quitting several times, but I completed the whole race and met my objectives for the day. The sense of personal power I experienced as I crossed the finish line stayed with me for the days and weeks that followed. Truthfully, this is an experience I continue to draw upon on a regular basis. When things get tough, I can think back to the fact that I made it out of the water that day.

This personal victory gave me the momentum to work even harder at conquering this chronic pain condition so that I could continue participating in this great sport that was giving me the opportunity to live the active, athletic life I craved. My health condition continued to improve as I was incredibly motivated to implement every possible solution I could find to manage my condition better.

I Caught the Triathlon Bug

I entered many triathlons over the next few years. Many times, my pre-race training involved almost no running. However, I was able to hold my own during the run on race day because of the hard work I was putting into strength and bike training. Once hooked on triathlon, I began aiming for longer distances. I completed my first Olympic distance triathlon (1,500 m swim, 40 km bike, and 10 km run) in 2011. That December, I told my friend MT about my crazy goal of doing a half-iron triathlon in 2012. The distances for the half-iron event are 1,900 m of swimming, 90 km of biking, and 21.1 km of running. Up until the Olympic distance, I was able to get away with very little running prior to race day. However, I knew those days were over if I had any hope of completing the half-iron distances inside the cut-off time. So I signed up for a half-marathon in the spring of 2012 to test out my ability to go the distance on the run. MT volunteered to run it with me.

In January, once my May half-marathon date was set, I decided to commit myself and actually register for a half-iron triathlon event. I wanted something as late in the summer as possible to give me a chance to (a) recover from the May half-marathon if I happened to get injured, and (b) improve my swimming and biking as much as possible. My online search revealed a few races in Ontario in late August and early September. For some reason, I was drawn to a Somersault Event in Ottawa on Labor Day weekend. The date had not been confirmed at that point, so I went back a few weeks later to check on registration. The date had been confirmed for September 1—I almost fell out of my chair. September 1 was my dad's birthday, and he was born and buried in Ottawa. I broke into tears as I signed up for the race on the spot. This was meant to be. I would dedicate this race to my dad. When he died in 2005, I was not doing well at all. I was always in pain and discomfort, stretching and rolling on my tennis ball on the floor. This would be my way of showing him I was doing so much better than the last time he saw me.

In the months to follow, I ran more per week than I probably had in my life, and certainly since my early twenties. I also ramped up my swim and bike workouts. Although the running volume was relatively high for me, I was conservative by anyone else's measures. I rarely exceeded two runs per week, often only doing one per week. That being said, I was doing lots of strength and yoga training in between swim, bike, and run workouts to protect myself from injury as much as possible.

There were a few setbacks.

Because of my tight hips and Achilles tendons, my longest

training run (and the longest run of my life to date) prior to the May half-marathon was 16 km. I had hoped to get close to 20 km before the event, but I had to settle with an injury-free 16 km. I had heard many times that it's better to be 10 percent undertrained than 1 percent over-trained, because a rested body will outperform a tired body that's bordering on injury. I continued to test and prove this theory to myself with just about every race I entered! I actually tended to be about 25 to 50 percent undertrained, at least from the running perspective. Nevertheless, I believed that I was better off making up for the lack of running with extra swimming and cycling, which worked my cardiovascular fitness without the excess strain on my joints and soft tissues.

I successfully completed the half-marathon in May, but the summer of 2012 was full of ups and downs from a health perspective. My newly embraced Health Champion approach was put to the test when I suffered symptoms indicative of potential heart trouble. Through research, asking questions, and finding the right team members, I was able to get to the bottom of the issue and overcome the challenges that were thrown at me. This is when it really became clear that new health challenges were opportunities to uncover new information that could result in becoming even healthier. I was able to complete a sprint distance and an Olympic distance race in preparation for my September 1 half-iron event, which I was ready to tackle and believed I could complete in a respectable time.

With the whole family along to cheer me on in Ottawa, we drove straight to the cemetery to say hi to my dad. Rod and I had a good cry as the girls arranged and rearranged the flowers on the grave and tried to cheer me up. All I could think of saying to my dad was, "I'm okay, Dad, see? I'm doing a half-iron triathlon tomorrow!"

The next day, with *Daddy* written in Sharpie marker on my left arm, I truly felt like my dad was there, pulling me through the water and directing the wind to blow from behind. I surprised myself with great swim and bike times, and had an exceptional first 16 km on the run. It was a bit of a struggle to finish the last 5 km with burning pain under my feet. However, dedicating my effort to my dad made it tolerable. Once again, I thought this was the ultimate. This was it. I had fulfilled my potential. I was so grateful for my family supporting me (Rod and the girls cheered for me through the entire 6 hours and 34 minutes), and for being as strong and healthy as I now was.

Over the next few months, a few of my triathlete colleagues, Rod, and even the kids raised the inevitable question: "So, are you going to do an IRONMAN triathlon next?" I have to say, it was tempting to at least dream about it. If I could jump from an Olympic distance to a half-iron distance, why couldn't I jump from half-iron to full IRONMAN? There were two parts of my brain sending me conflicting messages. The doubtful one said, "You can't do that. IRONMAN races are for mega-athletes. It's way too much for your fragile body. You could never run the marathon portion." But the other part of my brain was sheepishly interjecting now and then, saying, "Just maybe ...."

Not long after the seed was planted, I began to believe I might be able to complete a full distance triathlon. I set my sights on the 2013 Subaru IRONMAN Mont-Tremblant North American Championship. As soon as I hit the "send" button on my registration, I started to panic. What was I doing? I had just committed to doing an IRONMAN! And I put a significant amount of my family's money behind it! "Get the training manual out," I told myself. "You have to get serious." It's amazing how you're driven to do your workouts when you've signed up for something that seems so scary and impossible to your rational brain.

In May 2013 I suffered through my first marathon, which was part of my physical and mental preparation for the IRONMAN distances. Hip pain and plantar fasciitis surfaced during the marathon, leaving me with just over three months to deal with them in time for the August 18 IRONMAN event. With the help of advice from Jillian my strength trainer, Carm my chiropractor, and a few elite triathletes from our training club, I was able to get through most of the summer with just enough run training to think I might be able to cross the finish line. A good amount of the "running" involved the elliptical trainer and water running with a floating belt to limit the pounding on my feet and hips, but it all counted in my mind. It was looking doable until three weeks before the race, when it felt like I had pulled my calf muscle.

Let's just say I was presented with many opportunities to conquer adversity that summer. I remained focused on implementing what I knew was effective for optimizing my soft tissue function, and on identifying new approaches that might further enhance my condition. Just in time, I discovered IV electrolyte infusions and trigger point injections (both of these are covered in Chapter 10). Combined with everything else I was doing, these were the additional treatments I needed to get me to the start line believing there was a good chance I could complete the race.

With everything I had overcome to this point, I felt that no matter what the result of my IRONMAN attempt, my life was so much more rewarding and fulfilling than ever as a result of striving for it. It truly is about "the climb" and not about arriving somewhere. Einstein's statement comes to mind here: "The value of achievement is in the achieving."

On August 18, 2013, I showed up for the Subaru IRONMAN race in Mont-Tremblant, Quebec. Standing on the beach at the start line, the victory was mine. Finishing would be a bonus.

How Does It Feel to Complete an IRONMAN?

I imagine it feels different for everyone. But for someone

like me, who never thought she could get past running a few kilometers without getting injured, I would describe it as disbelief mixed with elation! I learned a lot about myself on August 18, 2013 at IRONMAN Mont-Tremblant. I now know I can drive myself further than I ever believed possible. If a goal is worthy, I will never listen to that little voice inside that says, "That's impossible; you can't do that."

As difficult as it was, as much discomfort as there was during the bike and run, when I heard the announcer call out, "Carole Staveley, YOU ARE AN IRONMAN" and the crowd going crazy, with my husband and kids yelling so loudly I could hear them above everyone else, it made all the pain and exhaustion disappear. One minute I'm thinking, "Never again, this is it, only one IRONMAN," and the next (after crossing the finish line) I'm thinking, "Where do I sign up for the next one?" Following is a summary of how the day went.

Race Day—Before the 7:00 a.m. Start

Although the logical part of my brain kept telling me that I should be nervous before the start, I was surprisingly calm. I had done everything I could to prepare my body for this, including the training, the chiropractor visits, the hydration, nutrition, etc. I was truly grateful to be a participant. I had nothing to lose. My only competition was the cut-off times. I had to finish the swim in less than 2 hours and 20 minutes, get off the bike before 5:30 p.m. (10.5 hours after race start), and come in from the run before midnight (a total of 17 hours). I also had a personal goal of completing it in less than 15 hours, but that was a bonus as far as I was concerned.

The scene on the beach was as powerful as I had imagined for all the months leading up to the event. There were 2,600 athletes including some of the world's best, along with 2,000 or more spectators on the beach. Royal Canadian Air Force jets flew above to salute us and the daunting challenge we were about to take on. There were cannon shots and fireworks to signal the start of each wave of athletes, mine being the "women 35+" wave. The forecast called for a beautiful warm and sunny day. The lake shimmered with the reflection of the newly risen sun and the Laurentian Mountains stood tall in the distance, adding to a feeling of awe and gratitude that was mounting within me.

The Swim

I positioned myself near the back of the pack to start the swim. With about six hundred women in the 35+ age group, most of whom could swim faster than me, I didn't want the pressure of having people at my heels trying to overtake me. One last round of high fives and hugs from Rod and the girls, then I was making my way into the water. All I could hear was the counting in my head that I use to keep myself focused. On every twelfth stroke, I would look toward the orange buoys marking the 3.8 km swim course. Next, the positive and upbeat lyrics from Will.i.am's "#thatPOWER" entered my head: "I'm loving every second, minute, hour, bigger, better, stronger, power ... I've got that power." I was incredibly relaxed, telling myself I've done this distance before. All went well, and I came out of the water in about 1 hour and 50 minutes, just as I expected and well within the 2 hour and 20 minute cutoff. Rod and the kids were there cheering for me, giving me extra energy in preparation for the bike portion.

The Bike

I started out with an upset stomach, but I tried to let it not bother me and had a really good first 1.5 hours ... until the wind started to pick up and the hills got bigger. Up to about 5 hours, I held my own, but then the pain started to set in—mainly in my butt, back, legs, and feet. I was starting to wonder how I could run a marathon after this. In addition, I had to make four port-o-potty stops because of the stomach upset. Finally, after about 7 hours (and within the cutoff time), I reached the transition area and gladly handed my bike over to a volunteer. Rod later told me he was surprised to see such a huge grin on my face after the long and grueling bike ride. Little did he know it was the overwhelming relief of getting my butt off the bike seat that was behind that big grin. For all I cared in that moment, they could have donated my bike to charity! In fact, running a marathon now seemed like a welcome activity.

The Run

With the help of an incredible volunteer chiropractor, my legs and feet felt a lot better after my 13-minute transition from the bike. Although I was still somewhat concerned about my body holding up for a full marathon, I told myself, "One step at a time." I figured I would run until I couldn't run anymore, and then I could always walk if I needed to. I truly surprised myself. Make no mistake; there was lots of discomfort, but nothing I couldn't overcome. Other than walking up some hills and taking a few breaks now and then (including two more port-o-potty stops), I ran the whole way! I kept checking my watch, knowing I would have to run most of it to make my sub-15 hour goal.

When I finally got to the last kilometer, I could hear the announcers at the finish line and see the lights and fireworks going off. My adrenaline kicked in and I found speed I really didn't know I had in me. That was the longest kilometer ever, but I finished strong. I heard my husband and kids screaming over the crowd, I turned to see them just a few steps from the finish line. Then I crossed and heard, "Carole Staveley, YOU ARE AN IRONMAN!" It is so difficult to describe the relief, disbelief, pure joy, and shock I felt in that moment.

The following few minutes after crossing the finish are a blur. I received my medal, had my finisher's photo taken, and searched for Rod and the kids. They were exhausted from the 18-hour day they had spent supporting me, giving me one hundred percent of their energy. Although cold, wet, and spent, I was the one with all the energy as we walked the kilometer or so back to our hotel room, still high from the IRONMAN experience.

My finish time was 14 hours and 47 minutes. It was a personal victory to show up at the start line. It is a feat beyond my wildest dreams to have completed it. It is my wish that others with chronic health conditions can find hope in my story, and never give up the search for solutions that can take them to the next level.

I wanted to share this experience with you, not to imply that everyone should have an IRONMAN triathlon on their goals list, but rather to give you the inspiration to imagine what you might be able to accomplish one day. If you can't walk a mile today, can you envision taking action toward walking that mile one day? How about a hundred meters by next month or next year? What actions can you begin to take toward becoming your own Health Champion, to make that goal seem realistic? Once you achieve your modest goal, the doors of your mind could open, and you might have the courage to think, "Just maybe I can take it a step further."

Getting Started in Triathlon

If my story in any way piques your interest in triathlon, I encourage you to look into it. There are so many great reasons to participate. Here are just a few:

- Signing up for races in advance gives you a goal to work toward. Entry fees are affordable, but the fact that you've committed money in advance increases the odds you'll train and show up.

- Like other individual sports, you're really just racing against yourself, which takes the pressure off. You can always look back and see how you did within your age group, and set goals that way, or you can simply set goals according to your individual time results.
- The cross-training between the three sports (swimming, cycling, and running) keeps things interesting and limits the impact on your body since there's only one impact sport out of the three.
- Event day is always inspiring, as you'll see top professionals, people showing up for their first-ever triathlon, disabled athletes, and everything in between. Everyone is there for their own personal reason, and it is a very supportive environment. Out on the race course, you'll often hear things like "keep it up" or "you're doing great, just a little further" being called out from one athlete to another.

Picking an Event

I put this section ahead of any training tips, because I think it's key to pick a target event first. Go online and search for "triathlons" in your area. You should see a number of them pop up. Triathlon has become a very popular sport in North America. What's interesting is that the fastest growth in the sport has come from the 40+ age groups. There are generally five types of triathlon distances:

1. Beginner—These are typically labeled "Try a Tri" or "Give it a Tri." Distances for each event vary, but generally, the swim distance is between 250 to 400 m (10 to 16 laps of a 25-m pool), the bike is 10 to 15 km, and the run is around 2.5 km.

2. Sprint distance—Again, there is some variation in the distances; however, the range is typically as follows: swim 500 to 750 m, bike 20 to 30 km, run 5 to 7.5 km.
3. Olympic distance—This one is set in stone, as it is the internationally recognized format for the Olympic triathlon event: 1,500 m swim, 40 km bike, and 10 km run.
4. Half-Iron distance (sometimes referred to as half-ironman or "70.3," which is the label used for events officially sanctioned by the World Triathlon Corporation)—Distances are 1,900 m swim, 90 km bike and 21.1 km run.
5. Full distance or IRONMAN (registered trademark of World Triathlon Corporation)—Distances are 3,800 m swim, 180 km bike, and 42.2 km run.

Whatever your current level of fitness, select a distance that is a stretch for you right now. If you can swim and bike but can't run or walk, many races will offer a "swim/bike" event. If swimming is not your thing, there will often be a duathlon (bike/run) option at the event. Even better, if you sign up for the triathlon event and change your mind on race day due to injury or nerves, the organizers can almost always accommodate a downgrade in your event.

And if those aren't enough options for you, many events will have a relay option. In other words, you show up as a team of three people, each one assigned to complete either the swim, bike, or run portion. It's pretty difficult to come up with solid excuses as to why you can't participate in a triathlon event. Now get on the computer and find the event that's right for you. Sign up and pay the money!

Setting Your Goals for the Event

As I mentioned earlier in the book, I had three clear goals for my first Sprint triathlon:

1. Don't get hurt.
2. Finish.
3. Don't be last in my age group

The first two were the goals that mattered most to me, and the third was a "nice to do." I would only know the outcome of this third goal after the fact, when the final race results were posted. You decide on what your goals are, aside from maybe just showing up and doing your best. As I became more experienced, I began setting time goals for myself for each part of the race, as well as overall time goals. This made it motivating because it allowed me to track my progress. If there is an event for which I don't feel quite prepared, I simply look at it as a "training event" without any specific time goals. Surprisingly, I ended up having a personal best time for one such race! Keep in mind that the result for your first race is always a personal best.

Equipment Needs

The basic equipment for triathlon training is pretty straightforward: a swimsuit, goggles, a bicycle, a helmet, and running shoes. However, there are several additional considerations, including the following.

A Wetsuit

For open-water swimming, I highly recommend the use of a wetsuit. There are important benefits to it like keeping you warmer and increasing your buoyancy. Its importance is heightened in cold water and for longer distance swims. However, there are some downsides, like (1) the constrained feeling takes some getting used to; (2) it can be challenging to pull off when you get out of the water; and (3) they're not cheap. Your swimming ability and your ability to tolerate cold should guide your decision about purchasing one. Note that some triathlon shops and race events offer rentals for a reasonable price. If available to you, this is a good option for your first race.

A Racing or Triathlon Bicycle

Many athletes participating in shorter distance events use whatever bicycle they have on hand. I used my "hybrid" bicycle, which looks like a mountain bike, with road tires on it for my first two Sprint Distance races. Once I committed to triathlons for the longer term, I purchased a good quality "road racing" bicycle. This is the bicycle I've stuck with to this day. Although the majority of participants in longer distance races are equipped with specially designed triathlon bicycles that can shave minutes off their time, I never saw the need to invest further. Choose a lightweight bicycle and ensure that it fits you properly. Once you move to a road or triathlon bicycle, please ensure you work with an expert to help you choose the bike design and size that is right for you. And it is critical to invest in a session with a bike fitter to have it adjusted to your body's biomechanics. Not only can this enhance your performance, but it can also reduce your risk of repetitive motion injuries over time.

A Heart Rate Monitor

As I learn more about the science of proper training, I realize that you have to practice different types of cardiovascular workouts in order to safely and effectively improve both your speed and endurance. You can't properly implement the different training approaches (high intensity intervals versus long distances at moderate intensity, for example) unless you have some measure of effort level, and heart rate is the most accessible and affordable way to measure this. For about $150 you can get a basic heart rate monitor. That's all I use. You can get really fancy and buy some in the $350-plus range, but unless you love technology, I don't advise it. They have many functions that you'll likely never use, and most need to be recharged regularly. For some of us that means it'll never be charged when you need it!

Cycling Shorts

As your distances increase on the bike, you'll want to own at least one pair of cycling shorts. The padding can increase the distances tolerated by your butt. However, I strongly advise that you try on a number of different models before buying them. I've had a few pairs with padding in the wrong places for my body, meaning I might have enjoyed the ride more with no padding at all. In the end, it's a trial and error process.

Running Socks

You'd be surprised what a difference the right socks can make. Everyone has their own advice on this, and I have to say I've tried many different types of socks. The ones I keep coming back to are the thicker, padded Thorlo® running socks. However, the majority of people swear by thinner socks in terms of preventing blisters. Again, you'll have to weigh the data and try them out for yourself before settling on your particular favorites.

Running Shoe Options

You'll see lots of information from shoe manufacturers detailing why their particular shoe models are better than others. However, I was told by a chiropractor who specializes in running technique that the choice in running shoes simply comes down to the user's comfort. The best thing to do is go to a running store with multiple shoe options, listen to the salesperson's input about key considerations, and try on as many styles as possible. Walk and run a bit in each, and base your decision on what feels good. In the end, it will be your biomechanics, muscle strength, and running technique that determine your risk of injury from running.

The additional options are endless, and as you move forward in your development as a triathlete, you'll discover additional tools and gadgets that can further enhance your training and race experiences. The most important thing is to get started with whatever you have. Now.

Your Training Plan

Obtaining some training direction from experts in the sport is critical to your success—both in terms of performance and injury prevention. Fortunately there are some high quality, affordable, and accessible training resources available. Following are some suggestions based on my experience.

Triathlon Training Guide

Do yourself a favor and buy a good triathlon training guide. The one I use is *Triathlete Magazine's Essential Week-by-Week Training Guide: Plans, Scheduling Tips, and Workout Goals for Triathletes of All Levels* by Matt Fitzgerald. It's an excellent guide for athletes of all levels. It's a little complicated to figure out at first, but once you get the hang of it, it's the best way to stay focused on what workouts to do when. Whether you complete all the workouts in the guide or not is irrelevant. It's just about having some direction from an experienced coach. It takes all the stress out of training. Every Sunday in training season, I would fit the week's workouts into my calendar, and it was done. Every day, I knew exactly what to do when. My only caution is that it does not include guidance around strength and flexibility training. Both are key to avoiding injuries, so you'll likely want to replace a few triathlon workouts with strength and flexibility training.

Triathlon Training Clubs

More and more of these are popping up all over the country, with the increasing popularity of triathlon. If you like the extra motivation and camaraderie that come with group training, this is a great option. Rod and I belong to the Canadian Cross Training Club, which we use mainly for our swim training.[31] They do offer regular training sessions for running, cycling, and yoga as well, which I would love to attend, but the logistics become complicated with work and kids! Swimming is the one discipline for which I need the most external motivation, so I sign up and put down the money for the swim sessions. With most of these training groups, you should be able to pick and choose which discipline(s) you wish to sign up for (swim, bike, and/or run), and how many times per week you want to join in.

Swimming

If you're not already a strong swimmer, I recommend joining a swimming group in your area. There are many Masters Swim programs across Canada and the US. Various clubs will have Masters Swim groups with objectives ranging from entering sanctioned swim competitions to triathlon preparation to simply encouraging each other to show up and work on strokes. Most clubs or groups will have a wide range of abilities within the group.

In my first season, I went from being the slowest in the slow lane to the second slowest in the slow lane by the end of the season ... yay! I'm still a member of the slow lane; however, depending on who shows up for the workout, I've been the fastest in that lane a few times. If you're not a very strong swimmer, try to find a group that is headed up by a highly competent coach, at minimum a national level competitive swimmer or

---

[31]C3Online.ca

ex-swimmer. This way, you'll get some good technique tips that will make your life easier down the road. If you can't swim at all, it's time to learn. Most local community centers offer very affordable adult "learn to swim" programs. Start there, with a goal to advance to a Masters Swim program.[32]

Cycling

A lot of people will tell you that in order to improve your cycling, you just have to put the miles in. In my experience, this is only partially true. You can't really improve without the mileage. However, your greatest improvements will come from implementing a cycling program that alternates between shorter, high intensity workouts and longer, lower intensity workouts. During the summer months, I will do my longer, lower intensity rides outside and will take the bike inside to do the higher intensity interval workouts. This is because it's so much easier to control the conditions when you're inside. You don't want to ramp up for a two-minute high intensity interval, only to run into a stop sign!

Having some direction and motivation for the high intensity rides is really valuable. I've invested in some video cycling classes called Spinervals by Coach Troy Jacobson. You can look into purchasing DVDs or downloads at spinervals.com. Look for the strength building series, and any other sessions that would indicate high intensity interval training. You can either do these on a stationary bike at home or at the gym, or you can buy a trainer for your bike—essentially a contraption that turns your bike into a stationary one. You can ask about these at any bike shop in your area. Another great option is to take part in some spinning classes at your local gym or spinning studio, just to mix things up and keep it interesting. You can make these

---

[32]Start here to find a Masters swim group in your area: usms.org/lmsc (US); and mymsc.ca/ClubList.jsp (Canada).

as high or low intensity as you want, depending on what your training goal is for that day.

Running

Running is both the most straightforward and the most complicated part of triathlon training for me. It's so straightforward, because all I have to do is put on a pair of running shoes and head out my front door to get my workout in. It's so complicated because, out of the three disciplines, it's the hardest on my body. My approach is to get away with the least amount of running possible while ensuring I can go the distance at my targeted race event. While the training plan might tell me to run twice a week or more, I rarely run more than once a week, and it's usually more like once every two weeks. I will substitute a strength workout, a bike workout, the elliptical trainer, or water running for that extra run I'm supposed to do. This approach has worked for me for the past five years. If running is not an issue for you, I am envious. I love the sense of freedom that comes with running.

If you're nervous about running, you have lots of options. Here are a few:

- At least for some of your run training sessions, substitute the elliptical trainer, or buy yourself a floating belt to do some water running. Show up on race day prepared to run, but walk at least some of it if you have to.
- Find an exercise physiologist, chiropractor, or running coach who can help you with your form and give you drills to do, which can reduce your risk of injury.
- Remember that strength and flexibility training are critical to allow your soft tissues and joints to tolerate the repetitive impact of running. Strong muscles are essentially shock absorbers for the joints.

Strength and Flexibility Training

As mentioned earlier, I can't emphasize enough the importance of a customized, progressive strength training program designed by a professional, ideally a Certified or Registered Exercise Physiologist. You don't need to sign up for multiple weekly sessions with this person. If you're concerned about the expense, I can tell you that the value is incomparable. What I can also tell you is that you really only need two or three sessions in your first month to get you started on the right track and to ensure you're doing the exercises properly. Then you can check in once a month or once every six weeks or so, with the goal of adjusting the program in accordance with the progress you're making. As you become stronger and more self-sufficient, you can further reduce the frequency of appointments as long as you are self-motivated enough to do your strength workouts regularly on your own. You can also increase your odds of following through with your workouts by enlisting your spouse, friends, or children to do them with you.

Yoga is another key component of my strength and flexibility program. My goal is to average one yoga class per week throughout the year. That means one or two per week in the winter and one or two per month in the summer. If you don't think you need the customized strength program, at the very least try and get to a few yoga classes per week. It will help you develop the strength and flexibility needed for your soft tissues to respond more favorably to your other training.

Be Flexible

In this case, I'm talking about your mind's flexibility. As you work toward improving your fitness to achieve whatever triathlon goal you've set for yourself, expect that you will run into challenges. Each challenge represents an opportunity to problem-solve and to learn about even more ways to improve your health and fitness. Remember that the real reward comes from the process of moving toward the goal. There are so many options open to you if something goes wrong during your training season. Look for what you *can* accomplish, not what you *can't*. If a triathlon proves to be too much this coming year, then step down to a swim-bike event or a duathlon. Or get some friends to join in on a relay event. Or maybe the goal this year is just learning to swim, with a longer-term goal of completing a triathlon in two or three years.

Involve Your Kids

If you have kids living at home, triathlon can be a great way to keep the family active and healthy while increasing your time spent together. Whether you sign up the kids for a kids-only triathlon and cheer them on, have them join you in a "Try a Tri" relay event if they're old enough, or have the whole family attend an event that caters to all ages so that everyone has their own event to race in, you can make any aspect of triathlon a family event.

Conclusion

I have presented you with much to think about when it comes to taking control of your health as you strive to fulfill your life purpose. As mentioned earlier, I'm not offering a magic cure, because I think we can all agree that doesn't exist. Whether your pain is physical, mental, or emotional, becoming the healthiest person you can be is a process. There is no end point. This is why being a Health Champion is so motivating and rewarding. It is a journey of constant learning and self-improvement. There is always a new "you" on the horizon, waiting to be discovered. There is the prospect of becoming a greater contributor to society through self-discovery and self-improvement. My wish for you is that you discover the gifts of becoming a Health Champion in order to live the most productive, fulfilling, and satisfying life possible, regardless of your limitations.

Erasing the pain might be your ultimate dream, and I encourage you to continue your pursuit of enhanced pain-reduction techniques. This is a part of the Health Champion approach. And when pain is managed effectively, your motivation to take on additional Health Champion behaviors like goal setting and implementing novel treatments can be greatly enhanced. However, I believe we get into trouble when pain reduction becomes the end point of our search. When the expectation of a pain-free life supersedes everything, there is a great risk of missing out on what life has to offer.

I believe that in many cases, there is a place for medications that can help reduce your pain—of any type. In my view, it can be a temporary fix to allow you to get through the day so you can find a more permanent solution to manage the pain. Morphine for a patient having recently suffered an amputation, anti-anxiety medicine for someone whose anxiety is crippling; these are truly necessary and humane applications of pain reduction. But pain medication should not be viewed as *the* solution. It's a tool to help you find the long-term approaches that will allow you to live your life fully, despite the existence of some pain. Dan Baker, Ph.D. and author of *What Happy People Know*, makes the point that "happiness is the result of engaging in life fully, even when it hurts."

Before you even think about giving up, can you look in the mirror and tell yourself you've turned over every stone; consulted with every person who could possibly point you in the right direction; followed through with and implemented every suggestion; researched and asked all the questions you can think of? Are you committed to pursuing your WHY and making the most of every day, while maintaining hope for a better tomorrow?

When you look back at the end of your days, regardless of the pain you've experienced in your life, will you truly be able to say, "I did everything in my power to live to my fullest potential, and I have made the greatest contribution possible."

Before thirteen years of *your* life pass you by, I urge you to recognize and harness the power that you have in your current state. If everything in your life came easily, you would never be able to discover just how high you can go. It is the adversity— the difficulties—that, if utilized properly, can provide the fuel to drive us to new heights. Until you feel that you are a fully fledged Health Champion, you can refer back to the 9 Steps in this book to ensure you're applying them wholeheartedly. Think of your WHY, set your goals, build and leverage your team, and see just how far you can go. And when you cross *your* finish line, be sure to send me your story. I'm cheering for you every step of the way.

References and Resources

Building the Health Champion Mindset

Dan Baker, *What Happy People Know: How the New Science of Happiness Can Change Your Life for the Better*, Rodale, 2003. This was one of the first self-help books I read after losing my dad in 2005. I wanted to be happy again. This book helped me realize that true happiness has nothing to do with laughing all day long. It's about accepting that everything in life comes to an end and learning to love every moment as it happens more than we mourn its loss.

Brené Brown, Ph.D., *The Gifts of Imperfection: Let Go of Who You Think You're Supposed to Be and Embrace Who You Are*, Hazelden, 2010.

Bruce Grierson, *What Makes Olga Run: The Mystery of the 90-Something Track Star, and What She Can Teach Us About Living Longer, Happier Lives*, Random House Canada, 2014. This book provides fascinating insights into the science of aging, as well as an illustration of practical, everyday application of this science. It can provide the guidance you need to set realistic yet motivating goals toward a healthier, more valuable, and more fulfilled life despite advancing in age.

Susan Jeffers, Ph.D. *Feel the Fear and Do It Anyway*, Ballantine Books, 2007. As you prepare to take action on your Health Champion journey, this book might offer you some additional direction on turning fear, indecision, and anger into power, action, and love.

Simon Sinek, *Start With Why: How Great Leaders Inspire Everyone to Take Action*, Penguin Group, 2009.

Building and Leveraging Your Health Champion Team

Dr. Manon Bolliger, *What Patients Don't Say If Doctors Don't Ask: The Mindful Patient-Doctor Relationship*, Influence Publishing, 2012. Dr. Bolliger provides insight into a holistic, win-win relationship that can exist between health professionals and patients. It might help you determine whether your health professionals are taking a "whole patient" approach to your health problems.

Dr. Anthony Galea, *The Real Secret to Optimal Health*, Burman Books, 2013. This is a pretty comprehensive book that takes you through many steps to optimize your health. It can also serve as a useful resource to help you formulate questions to ask health professionals.

Susan Jeffers, Ph.D. *Feel the Fear and Do It Anyway*. Ballantine Books, 2007. In particular, Chapter 6 can be helpful for dealing with family members and friends who aren't supportive.

Todd Kashdan's insights on the science behind creating an enjoyable, meaningful life can help you identify who you want to include in your social network: toddkashdan.com.

Money Crashers. A good basic guide to budgeting, to help you identify how you could build your Health Champion fund: moneycrashers.com/how-to-make-a-budget.

Persevering

Carole Staveley, *Not Lying Down: How I Conquered Years of Pain to Triumph at the Finish Line*, Staveley Enterprises Inc., 2014. I wrote my first book primarily as my personal story from chronic pain sufferer to IRONMAN finisher, chronicled in greater detail than the examples given in this book. It also includes the story of how I overcame infertility. If you like personal stories, you might find some extra inspiration in this one.

carolestaveley.com. Feel free to review my blog posts for additional insights and motivation to reach higher and take on the challenges that stand in the way of reaching your potential. You can also check out my life coaching and other services on the site.

Erik Weihenmayer and Paul Stoltz, *The Adversity Advantage: Turning Everyday Struggles into Everyday Greatness*, Simon and Schuster, 2010. This book makes you think differently about the adversities you face in your everyday life. Instead of letting these challenges defeat you, you can take them on and use them as fuel to make you better and drive you further. If a blind man can climb the seven highest mountains in the world, what could you achieve by harnessing the power of adversities you encounter on a daily basis?

My "Believe" Playlist

Setting criteria for acquiring songs that have inspiring words, meaning, and musical arrangements, I've carefully selected fifty-two songs in four years of searching. I hope some of these will resonate for you and will help you through some of your more challenging moments.

- "Set Fire to the Rain" ADELE
- "Thank You" Alanis Morissette
- "Marching On" The Alarm
- "Spirit Of '76" The Alarm
- "The Stand" The Alarm
- "Where Were You Hiding When the Storm Broke" The Alarm
- "Keep Your Head Up" Andy Grammer
- "Hall of Fame" Andy Wanted
- "Pompeii" Bastille
- "Stand By Me" Ben E. King
- "I Love Myself Today" Bif Naked
- "Get Up, Stand Up" Bob Marley
- "It's My Life" Bon Jovi
- "Born to Run" Bruce Springsteen
- "Ain't No Rest for the Wicked" Cage the Elephant
- "Fighter" Christina Aguilera
- "Tubthumping" Chumbawamba
- "Inner Ninja" Classified
- "Rather Be" Clean Bandit
- "Skyscraper" Demi Lovato
- "Unbelievable" EMF
- "A Little Party Never Killed Nobody" Fergie, Q-Tip & GoonRock
- "Some Nights" Fun
- "Carry On" Fun

- "I Will Survive" Gloria Gaynor
- "Good Riddance (Time of Your Life)" Green Day
- "Know Your Enemy" Green Day
- "The Fighter" Gym Class Heroes
- "Anything" Hedley
- "On Top of the World" Imagine Dragons
- "What a Feeling" Irene Cara
- "Right Here Right Now" Jesus Jones
- "The Middle" Jimmy Eat World
- "Don't Stop Believin'" Journey
- "Born This Way" Lady GaGa
- "The Edge of Glory" Lady GaGa
- "Ain't No Mountain High Enough" Marvin Gaye & Tammi Terrell
- "Live Like a Warrior" Matisyahu
- "The Climb" Miley Cyrus
- "Shellshock" New Order
- "You Get What You Give" New Radicals
- "If Today Was Your Last Day" Nickelback
- "Feel This Moment" Pitbull
- "What I Wouldn't Do" Serena Ryder
- "Light Up" Single Ish
- "I'm Free" The Soup Dragons & Junior Reid
- "Eye of the Tiger" Survivor
- "Beautiful Day" U2
- "Two Hearts Beat As One" U2
- "#That Power" Will.i.am
- "Only You" Yaz
- "Wavin' Flag" Young Artists for Haiti

Covering All the Health Champion Principles

Inner Victory™ *e-Book of Health Champions*. You can download this inspiring e-book of Health Champion stories on my website at carolestaveley.com. Each personal story demonstrates the application of at least some of the 9 Steps shared in this book, resulting in better life outcomes for those individuals. I encourage you to download it, allow the stories to motivate you, and share it with others who could benefit from it.

Inner Victory™ *Health Champion Workbooks*. Also found on my website, carolestaveley.com, these workbooks will help you apply some of the most critical steps in becoming your own Health Champion, conquering your pain, and living life to the fullest.

Chronic Pain/Fibromyalgia

Clair Davies, NCTMB, *The Trigger Point Therapy Workbook* (Second Edition). New Harbinger Publications Inc. 2004. This can help you understand where the key trigger points are and guide your discussions with the right health professionals.

Fibromyalgia Patient Handbook. This is a helpful and succinct handbook from the American Chronic Pain Association to get you started down the road of identifying and managing the symptoms of fibromyalgia. theacpa.org/uploads/FibroHandbook.pdf.

Devin J. Starlanyl, Ph.D. *Fibromyalgia (FMS) and Chronic Myofascial Pain (CMP) Information for Patients and*

Supporters. This medical handout from 2012 on chronic myofascial pain was really useful in helping me understand my condition at a deeper level and offered several additional modalities to try myself or ask my health professionals about: homepages.sover. net/~devstar/myopain.htm.

Triathlon Training

Matt Fitzgerald, *Triathlete Magazine's Essential Week-by-Week Training Guide: Plans, Scheduling Tips, and Workout Goals for Triathletes of All Levels*, Warner Wellness Inc., 2006. This is the guide I used to train for both my half-iron distance and IRONMAN races. Although I made many adjustments to the recommended program, it was indispensable in focusing my training efforts on a weekly and daily basis. If you're interested in a triathlon of any distance, I highly recommend this book to help you with your training plan. Whether your goal is just to finish or to win the event outright, there is a program for every level. The only thing it doesn't emphasize is that most of us need to do strength and flexibility training in addition to the swim, bike, and run workouts.

Spinervals Cycling. Coach Troy's Spinervals cycling workouts are at spinervals.com. If you own a stationary bike or you're thinking of setting up a trainer to make use of your real bike during bad weather, you seriously need to consider buying some video training sessions. Coach Troy's training programs keep me motivated and force me to push harder than if left to my own devices. You can order DVDs or downloads from the Spinervals website.

Author Biography

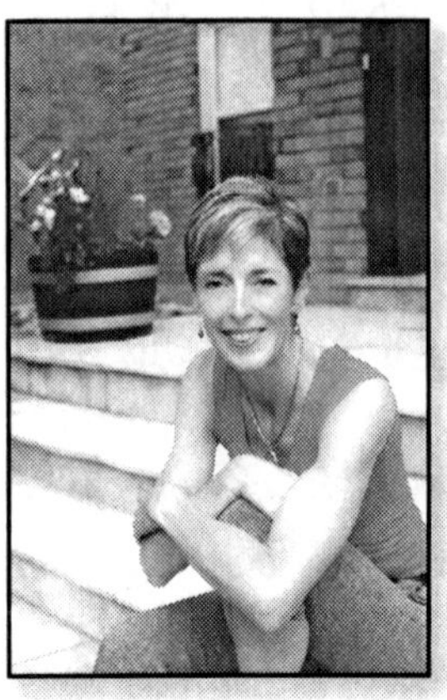

For thirteen years, Carole Staveley struggled against the debilitating pain and stiffness of chronic myofascial pain syndrome to maintain the active lifestyle she cherished and to stay fully engaged in her children's lives. Her breakthrough in the search for answers and relief came when she understood the need to take charge and seek out the right resources within and outside the medical community—a lesson she had already learned while addressing her infertility challenge. With nutritional changes, strength training, and other holistic treatment approaches, her chronic pain condition improved dramatically. Her first book, *Not Lying Down* (2014), details the story of how Carole won the battle against chronic myofascial pain syndrome to triumph at the finish line of an IRONMAN triathlon. This drove Carole to develop her 9 Step Health Champion system to help others overcome health challenges in a targeted and efficient manner. After a twenty-year career in the pharmaceuticals industry, Carole Staveley has embarked on a mission to empower others to take control of their health and become their own Health Champions.

Carole is President of Inner Victory Coaching, an organization focused on empowering individuals to take control of their health by providing educational publications and programs, including seminars, workshops, and coaching. She lives in Woodbridge, Ontario with her husband of twenty-three years and their two daughters.

Carole Staveley
Author ~ Speaker ~ Wellness Coach
President, Inner Victory Coaching

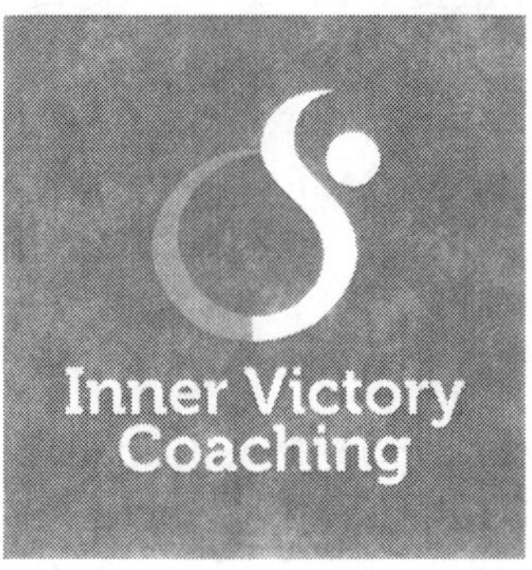

Carole's Previous Book

Not Lying Down: How I Conquered Years of Pain to Triumph at the Finish Line is available on Amazon and in ebook formats Kindle and Kobo.

Inner Victory Coaching—What We Do

Inner Victory Coaching, a company founded as a result of Carole's personal Health Champion journey, offers corporate and individual services aimed at empowering people to take control of their health. The Inner Victory 9—Step approach to becoming your own Health Champion underpins our workplace workshops, seminars, and health risk assessment programs. Additionally, we create personalized Victory Plans for individuals seeking coaching support to pursue their health goals and achieve their full potential. Our programs are based on the 9 Steps presented in this book, and built upon proven behavioral change systems and principles of human motivation.

Carole and Inner Victory Coaching in the Media

- Global TV interview with Rosey Edeh, 2014
- Monthly segments on Rogers TV Daytime, York Region, 2014-2015
- Rogers TV Daytime, Toronto, 2014
- Pain Revolution Radio with Dr. Peter Abaci, San Francisco, CA

Sample Speaking Engagements

- The Conference Board of Canada's Better Workplace Conference 2014, Calgary, Alberta
- Blissdom Conference, Mississauga, 2014
- Verity Club, Toronto, 2014
- ZoomerShow, Toronto, 2014
- Educational Seminar—The Big Carrot Natural Food Market, 2015, Toronto, Ontario

Check out www.carolestaveley.com and subscribe to the Inner Victory Coaching monthly newsletter

Connect Through Social Media

Youtube: youtube.com/user/CaroleStaveley
Facebook: CaroleStaveleyInnerVictoryCoaching
Twitter: @CaroleStaveley
LinkedIn: Carole Staveley

If you want to get on the path to becoming a published author
with Influence Publishing please go to
www.InfluencePublishing.com

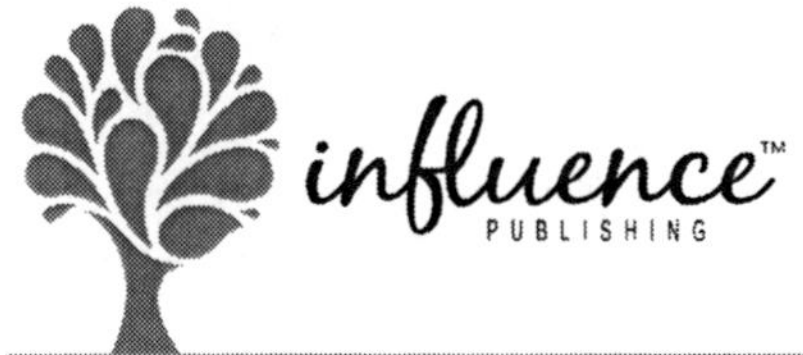

More information on our other titles and how to submit your
own proposal can be found at
www.InfluencePublishing.com

CPSIA information can be obtained at www.ICGtesting.com
Printed in the USA
LVOW07s0418300415

436680LV00004B/32/P